Classic Presentations and
Rapid Review for the USMLE, Step 2

Classic Presentations and
Rapid Review for the USMLE, Step 2

Theodore X. O'Connell, M.D.
Resident Physician
Department of Family Medicine
Santa Monica-UCLA Medical Center
Susan L. Taylor, M.D.
Resident Physician
Department of Family Medicine
Santa Monica-UCLA Medical Center
Sergio Huerta, M.D.
Resident Physician
Department of Surgery
University of California, Irvine
UCI Medical Center
Aamer H. Jamali, M.D.
Resident Physician
Department of Internal Medicine
Stanford University Medical Center

Edited by:

Theodore X. O'Connell, M.D.
Susan L. Taylor, M.D.
Kurt E. Johnson, Ph. D.

J&S

J&S Publishing Company Inc., Alexandria, Virginia

J&S

Composition and Layout: Ronald C. Bohn, Ph.D.
Cover Design: Theodore X. O'Connell, M.D. and Kurt E. Johnson, Ph.D.
Editorial Supervision: Kurt E. Johnson, Ph. D.
Printing Supervisor: Robert Perotti, Jr.
Printing: Goodway Graphics of Virginia, Inc., Springfield, VA

Library of Congress Catalog Card Number 98-066122

ISBN 1-888308-05-2

Table of Contents

Preface

Now that you have all passed the USMLE, Step 1, you will be glad to hear that the context and format of Step 2 test questions are similar to those in Step 1. All items are "single best answer", although some of the items contain more than five answers. As you probably remember, about 50% of the questions in Step 1 take the form of a clinical vignette. The key difference between Step 1 and Step 2 is that more than 90% of the Step 2 questions are in the format of clinical vignettes. This is the reason that we developed the "Classic Presentation" style in our book. Our clinical vignettes describe the "classic presentation" of a disease or clinical problem. By presenting the material this way, we hope to paint a picture for you of the most common presentations of diseases. Therefore, in as many subjects as possible, we begin the section by giving a classic presentation of the disease in question. The classic presentation is followed by other information about the disease which we deemed pertinent, such as etiology, prevalence, diagnosis, differential diagnoses, and treatment.

The primary goal of this book is to provide the basic information that is needed to do well on the USMLE, Step 2. We also hope that by painting pictures of classic presentation of illnesses, we will be helping with a lifetime of learning. If you are better able to remember how a disease typically presents, you will be better able to serve your patients.

Studying for Step 2 of the USMLE should begin early and be an active process. Keep in mind that you should be studying to become a great physician, not merely to pass an examination. Ideally, your studying should begin at the beginning of the third year of medical school. Make it a point to see as many of your own patients as possible and be active in their care. By seeing patients, you will begin to form an idea of real-life classic presentations of illnesses. Rather than waiting for a resident or attending to tell you what to do, try to come up with your own diagnosis and treatment plan. By being an active member of your patient's health care team, you will be more likely learn about important diseases and will be more able to retain this information. It is also important to read about your patients' illnesses, as this will provide you with a greater understanding of the pathogenesis and treatment of the disease. We recommend that you use this book as a supplement to the recommended textbooks during your third year clerkships. This book can be used to focus on the important details which may be obscured in a more detailed, more comprehensive textbook.

In studying specifically for Step 2 of the USMLE, we recommend that you start reading this book about three weeks prior to the examination. Try to finish a chapter every day, and when you finish we recommend that you review the chapters in which you felt "weaker" a second time. This should leave about one week before the examination. During this time we recommend that you try doing some practice questions. We definitely recommend the sample questions and other materials provided by the USMLE with your application. These questions most closely resemble the real test items. There are also many review books available which consist solely of questions with explained answers that may help you to feel more comfortable with the style of test questions. Any problem areas should be studied again in this review book.

Of course, some of you will have less time than this to prepare for the examination. We recommend that you try to read as much of this book as possible, but if time is scarce, you should concentrate on the classic presentations (the first bullet of most subjects) and at least utilize the review materials provided by the NBME.

The passing scores vary slightly from year to year but are usually in the 170-180 range. This corresponds to answering 55-65% of the items correctly. Remember, there is no penalty for guessing on this exam. Do not leave answers blank.

We strongly recommend that you try to relax as much as possible the day before the examination. Though extra studying may help, it is likely to make you more anxious. Try to do something that will take your mind off the examination. Get some exercise, go to the movies, or have a nice dinner.

Items that should be taken to the examination include your USMLE admission ticket, a valid photo I.D., a sweater or sweatshirt, and snacks that can be eaten quietly to be considerate to your neighboring test-takers. Leave computers, calculators, music players, digital wrist watches, pagers, cell phones, and other electronic communication devices at home. Increased concerns about security of examination material precludes having such devices in the examination setting.

We hope that this book helps you to do your best on the examination. Good luck on the test and with the rest of your medical career.

Theodore X. O'Connell, M.D.
Susan L. Taylor, M.D.
Sergio Huerta, M.D.
Aamer H. Jamali, M.D.
January, 1999

Acknowledgements

The authors would like to thank Dan O'Connell and Kevin Dick for their hard work in the proofreading of the manuscript. Thanks also to Mike Shane for generously allowing us to use his computer to work on this project and for helping with our many computer questions. Molly Prindiville was likewise generous in allowing the use of her computer to help us complete this project. The faculty and staff of the UCLA School of Medicine deserve a very warm thanks for all of their teaching, support, and help during our four years there. Finally, we wish to thank Kurt E. Johnson, Ph. D., our publisher at J&S Publishing Company Inc., for his support and editorial contributions throughout the writing of this book.

Disclaimer

The clinical information presented in this book is accurate for the purposes of review for licensure examinations but in no way should be used to treat patients or substituted for modern clinical training. Proper diagnosis and treatment of patients requires comprehensive evaluation of all symptoms, careful monitoring for adverse responses to treatment and assessment of the long-term consequences of therapeutic intervention.

Suggestions for Improvement

The authors of this book aim to make all of the information that has been presented as accurate and up-to-date as possible. Since this book is written for students, we would appreciate any feedback that you would like to give. In an effort to keep the book updated, we would like to hear your suggestions for future editions of this book. If there were areas which were heavily tested on the USMLE or if there were areas that were not covered in sufficient detail in this book, please let us know. If there are errors in the book or topics that are no longer clinically applicable, please let us know so that we can continue to improve this book for future students. If your suggestions are used in future editions of this book, we will thank you by name in the next edition of this book. Please forward all suggestions to us through our publisher:

Classic Presentations Authors
c/o J & S Publishing Company, Inc.
1300 Bishop Lane
Alexandria, VA 22302, USA
Phone 703-823-9833
Fax 703-823-9834
e-mail jandspub@ix.netcom.com
http://www.jandspub.com

Chapter 1

PEDIATRICS

Theodore X. O'Connell, M.D.

INFANCY

Apgar Scores

Points Awarded			
	0	**1**	**2**
Appearance	Central cyanosis	Peripheral cyanosis	Completely pink
Pulse	Absent	<100 bpm	>100 bpm
Grimace/ irritability	No response	Grimace	Cough or sneeze
Activity	No muscle tone	Some flexion	Normal flexion
Respirations	Absent	Irregular/ weak cry	Regular/ strong cry

- The 1-minute score indicates the infant's well-being; <3 implies asphyxia.
- The 5-minute score indicates continued well-being or decline. If the score is <7 at 5 minutes, it should continue to be taken every 5 minutes.

Cerebral Palsy
- Cerebral palsy (CP) is defined as a deficit restricted to the motor cortex, often due to a perinatal hypoxic insult, although it is frequently idiopathic.
- CP is a nonprogressive disorder of movement and posture secondary to brain injury or malformation.
- Etiology: About 60% prenatal, 30% perinatal, 10% postnatal.
- Sixty percent of patients with CP also have mental retardation, which is a secondary diagnosis.

Hyperbilirubinemia
- Unconjugated hyperbilirubinemia is the most common type of hyperbilirubinemia in the neonate.
- It is caused by an increased breakdown of blood from polycythemia or bruises, hemolysis due to blood group incompatibility, or insufficient glucuronyl transferase.
- Treat with phototherapy. Exchange transfusion can sometimes be used. Also treat any underlying disease.
- Elevated conjugated bilirubin levels are seen in biliary atresia.

Kernicterus
- Kernicterus results from indirect bilirubin deposition in the basal ganglia.
- This condition causes choreoathetoid cerebral palsy, deafness, mental retardation, and seizures.
- It is an irreversible condition that is a complication of hyperbilirubinemia.

Respiratory Distress Syndrome
- *CLASSIC PRESENTATION*: A premature infant with cyanosis, grunting respirations, and retractions.
- Respiratory distress syndrome is also referred to as hyaline membrane disease.
- This is a pulmonary disease associated with prematurity. It is caused by surfactant deficiency.
- Treat with surfactant. Sometimes intubation is necessary.

Choanal Atresia
- *CLASSIC PRESENTATION*: A newborn infant with failure to breathe and cyanosis that is alleviated when the infant cries.
- Choanal atresia is caused by a congenital membranous or bony septum between the nose and pharynx.
- Most newborns breathe effectively only through their noses, so the obstruction is bypassed when they cry and thus breathe through their mouths.
- Those infants that are able to mouth breathe become cyanotic when they try to feed.
- Treat with surgical repair.

Congenital Adrenal Hyperplasia (CAH)
- 21-hydroxylase deficiency and 11-hydroxylase deficiency account for most cases of CAH.
- 21-hydroxylase deficiency accounts for 90% of cases.
- Female infants with 21-hydroxylase deficiency are born with ambiguous genitalia while male infants have no visible abnormalities.
- Infants are classically acidotic, hyponatremic, and hyperkalemic.
- 11-hydroxylase deficiency accounts for 5% of the cases of CAH.
- These infants are classically hypertensive and hypokalemic

Breast-Feeding
- Fluoride and iron supplements should be given to the infant starting at six months.
- Vitamin D supplementation to the infant is recommended.
- Vitamin B supplementation to the infant is recommended if the mother is a vegetarian.

- Colostrum is the first secretion produced by the breast during late pregnancy and soon after delivery. Colostrum has more protein and vitamins than breast milk, and less fat. It is especially rich in secretory IgA and other immune substances.

Sudden Infant Death Syndrome (SIDS)

- The leading cause of death in the 1- to 12-month age group.
- Diagnosed by exclusion when death of an infant occurs unexpectedly and without explanation.
- Most common between 2 to 5 months and is more common in males.
- Risk factors include low socioeconomic status, low birth weight, positive family history of SIDS, infants of substance-abusing mothers, and infants put to sleep on their abdomens.
- Incidence has declined by educating parents to put infants to sleep on their backs and remove fluffy, loose bedding from the crib.

DEVELOPMENT

Developmental Milestones

Age	Gross motor skills	Fine motor skills	Language
6 months	Sits up	Transfers	Uses nonspecific vowel sounds, will soon begin babbling
1 year	Takes first step	Drinks from cup	Uses a few words
2 years	Climbs up and down stairs with immature gait, runs	Stacks 6-8 cubes	Uses 2-word phrases
3 years	Rides tricycle, climbs up stairs with mature gait	Able to wiggle thumb	Uses 3-word phrases
4 years	Hops, goes down stairs with mature gait	Draws person with 3 body parts	Able to define 5 words
5 years	Skips	Draws person with 6 body parts	Able to define 7 words

Linguistic Developmental Issues
- Linguistic development is the best predictor of future intelligence.
- When considering deficiency of linguistic development, one must first consider that the child may have a hearing problem.
- Also consider the possibility of mental retardation, autism, or environmental factors such as lack of sensory input.

Puberty
- The signs of puberty are listed below in order of appearance.
- Girls: breast buds, appearance of pubic hair, growth spurt, menarche.
- Boys: testicular enlargement, appearance of pubic hair, growth spurt.

Nocturnal Enuresis
- Nocturnal enuresis is defined as nighttime bedwetting.
- It is more common in males and there is often a positive family history.
- Fifteen percent prevalence at 5 years, 3% at 12 years.
- Intervention should be considered at 5 to 6 years.
- Obtain a detailed history and physical, urinalysis, and urine culture.
- A small bladder capacity is a common finding.
- Treat with motivational counseling, bladder training, enuresis alarms, and, occasionally medications.

Scoliosis
- *CLASSIC PRESENTATION:* An adolescent female with asymptomatic, asymmetric shoulder levels and one side of the posterior chest elevated upon bending forward.

INFECTIOUS DISEASES

Pneumonia, Meningitis, and Sepsis

Age	Causative Organism(s)	Antibiotic Therapy
Neonatal	Group B *Streptococcus* *E. coli* *Listeria*	ampicillin and gentamicin
4-8 weeks	Both groups	ampicillin and cefotaxime
>8 weeks	*Streptococcus pneumoniae* *Neisseria meningitidis* *Haemophilus influenzae*	cefotaxime

- Meningitis is most often seen in the first 30 days of life.
- In cases of *H. influenzae* meningitis, rifampin should be given to household contacts <4 years old for prophylaxis.
- All children with bacterial meningitis should have a hearing assessment since deafness is a common sequelae.
- Sensorineural hearing loss is generally noted early in the course of bacterial meningitis (especially with *S. pneumoniae*) and occurs despite prompt initiation of antimicrobial therapy. Some authorities advocate the use of steroids to decrease the incidence of hearing loss.

Neonatal Sepsis
- *CLASSIC PRESENTATION*: An infant with nonspecific symptoms such as poor feeding, irritability, apnea, abdominal distension, and temperature instability.
- Admit to hospital.
- Work-up includes CBC, as well as blood and urine cultures. Chest x-ray and lumbar puncture should be considered.
- Treat empirically with ampicillin and gentamicin.

Chlamydial Pneumonia
- *CLASSIC PRESENTATION*: A child several weeks-old with a history of conjunctivitis who now has a dry staccato cough, tachypnea, bilateral inspiratory crackles, and slight expiratory wheezing. Bilateral pneumonia is present on chest x-ray and eosinophilia seen on differential blood count.
- Chlamydial pneumonia is often seen at 1 to 3 months in an infant delivered vaginally.
- Fifty percent have had previous conjunctivitis.
- Inclusion bodies may be seen on Giemsa stain of pus from the eye.
- Treat with erythromycin.

Mycoplasma Pneumonia
- *CLASSIC PRESENTATION*: An adolescent with fever, malaise, sore throat, and cough. Note that these symptoms may be similar to mononucleosis.
- It is the leading cause of pneumonia in adolescence.
- Perihilar and lower lobe infiltration is seen on chest x-ray.
- Treat with erythromycin.

Strep Throat
- *CLASSIC PRESENTATION*: An individual with palatal petechiae, exudative tonsils, fever, and anterior cervical lymphadenopathy.
- If left untreated, strep may result in rheumatic heart disease (most commonly mitral stenosis).

- Strep infection may also result in scarlet fever, which manifests as a sandpaper rash.
- Poststreptococcal glomerulonephritis may appear even in cases that have been treated properly.
- The treatment of choice is penicillin.

Otitis Media
- *CLASSIC PRESENTATION*: A young child with fever, irritability, and a bulging, red tympanic membrane which is immobile with insufflation.
- Bugs: *S. pneumoniae*, nontypable *H. influenzae*, *Moraxella catarrhalis*.
- Treat with amoxicillin or amoxicillin/clavulanic acid.

Acute Sinusitis
- *CLASSIC PRESENTATION*: A child with 3 to 5 days of fever, purulent nasal discharge, dry cough, and pain to palpation over sinuses.
- Bugs: same as otitis media.
- Acute sinusitis has the same treatment as otitis media except that sinusitis must be treated longer.
- Also consider obstruction or foreign body as a cause of sinusitis.

Otitis Externa
- *CLASSIC PRESENTATION*: A young child with pus and redness in the external auditory meatus, which is also exquisitely tender.
- *Pseudomonas* and *Staphylococcus* are the most common organisms.

Urinary Tract Infection (UTI)
- *E. coli* is the most common organism causing UTI.
- *Proteus* infection is associated with increased urinary pH and staghorn calculi.
- UTI must be considered as the cause of an unexplained fever in a young child.

Mononucleosis
- *CLASSIC PRESENTATION*: An adolescent or young adult with fever, pharyngitis, lymphadenopathy, and splenomegaly whose Monospot test is positive.
- Mononucleosis is caused by the Epstein-Barr virus.
- It is usually treated symptomatically.
- A rare complication of mononucleosis is splenic rupture, so patients are advised to avoid contact sports until they are fully recovered.

Cat Scratch Disease
- *CLASSIC PRESENTATION*: A child with tender, fluctuant axillary or cervical lymph nodes and low-grade fever after playing with kittens.

- Caused by *Bartonella henselae*.

Infantile Botulism
- *CLASSIC PRESENTATION*: A previously healthy child with the sudden onset of lethargy, poor feeding, constipation, and generalized weakness. There may be a history of honey ingestion and there may be evidence of bulging, spoiled canned foods in the home.
- Caused by *Clostridium botulinum*.
- This is an emergency.

Orbital vs. Periorbital Cellulitis
- Both types of cellulitis show fever, eyelid swelling, redness of the eye, and leukocytosis.
- Orbital cellulitis exhibits proptosis and limitation of extraocular mobility.
- Orbital cellulitis is an emergency and requires hospitalization and IV antibiotics.

Osteomyelitis
- Osteomyelitis occurs most frequently in the long bones of the lower extremities in children.
- The metaphysis is most frequently involved.
- *Staphylococcus* and *Streptococcus* account for most cases of osteomyelitis.
- *Salmonella* is common in patients with sickle cell anemia.
- *Pseudomonas* is the likely species when one receives a puncture wound that penetrates the sole of a shoe.
- About 50% of cases will present with a history of minor trauma.
- Symptoms of osteomyelitis include fever, localized bone tenderness, swelling, redness, and warmth.
- Diagnosis is usually made with a bone scan.
- Radiographs lag behind the clinical course by about 10 days.
- IV antibiotic therapy with staphylococcal coverage (oxacillin) for about 4 weeks is the usual treatment, unless a Gram-negative organism is suspected.

Febrile Seizures
- *CLASSIC PRESENTATION*: A young child who presents with generalized tonic-clonic seizure activity and a fever.
- Febrile seizures occur most commonly between 6 months and 6 years.
- There are no long-term sequelae.
- Before diagnosing febrile seizures, meningitis must be ruled out.
- Treatment is antipyretic therapy with acetaminophen.

Chronic Granulomatous Disease (CGD)

● *CLASSIC PRESENTATION*: A young child recurrent severe infection.
● These patients are prone to infection by catalase-producing organisms such as *Staphylococcus aureus*, fungi, and Gram-negative bacilli.
● CGD is due to a deficiency in NADPH oxidase.
● Diagnosed with nitroblue tetrazolium (NBT) test (think: CGD=NBT).*

Guillain-Barré Syndrome

● *CLASSIC PRESENTATION*: Progressive, symmetric motor weakness, areflexia, and autonomic instability in an individual with a history of infection (often respiratory) in the several weeks preceding the clinical onset of this syndrome.
● Symptoms classically begin 2 weeks after a viral infection and start in the distal muscles of the legs.
● Therapy is usually supportive but may require steroids or assisted ventilation.

Reye's Syndrome

● *CLASSIC PRESENTATION*: A child who is irritable, withdrawn, vomiting, and has an altered mental status who was treated several days earlier with aspirin for a fever.
● Reye's syndrome is commonly associated with varicella or viral influenza.
● Encephalopathy and acute liver dysfunction are the hallmarks of Reye's syndrome.
● Treatment is supportive.

*Thanks to Lee Miller for this gem.

RESPIRATORY DISTRESS

Respiratory Distress Syndrome (RDS) (Hyaline Membrane Disease)

● *CLASSIC PRESENTATION*: A preterm infant with tachypnea, grunting, nasal flaring, chest retractions, and cyanosis in the first 3 hours of life. Physical examination reveals decreased air entry on auscultation. A ground-glass pattern and atelectasis are seen on chest radiographs. Arterial blood gas shows hypoxia, hypercarbia, and metabolic acidosis.
● RDS is caused by a deficiency in pulmonary surfactant due to immaturity of lungs.
● There is an increased risk of RDS with male sex, delivery by caesarean section, or maternal gestational diabetes.
● There is an decreased risk of RDS with maternal hypertension, placental disruption, or maternal narcotic addiction (these all are things that have already stressed the infant).

- Treatment consists of surfactant replacement therapy and oxygen.
- Administration of corticosteroids to the mother 48 hours before delivery can accelerate the production of fetal lung surfactant.

Diaphragmatic Hernia

- *CLASSIC PRESENTATION*: A neonate with severe respiratory distress, cyanosis, and dyspnea shortly after birth. Physical examination reveals a scaphoid abdomen and diminished breath sounds on the affected side. Chest x-ray shows air-filled bowel in the thorax.
- Diaphragmatic hernia is caused failure of closure of the (most often the left) pleuroperitoneal canal, leaving a patent foramen (of Bochdalek) through which by abdominal contents are displaced into the thoracic cavity.
- There is ipsilateral pulmonary hypoplasia from compression of lung by abdominal contents.
- Treat diaphragmatic hernia with intubation, oxygenation, GI decompression, acid-base correction, and surgical removal of abdominal contents from the thorax with repair of the hernia.

Bronchiolitis

- *CLASSIC PRESENTATION*: A child less than 2 years old with mild upper respiratory tract symptoms and fever for several days, followed by lower respiratory tract involvement, paroxysmal cough, wheezing, tachypnea, dyspnea, irritability, and decreased appetite.
- The peak incidence of bronchiolitis is 6 months of age.
- The leading cause is respiratory syncytial virus (RSV).
- Treat severe cases with ribavirin or RSV immune globulin and supportive care.

Croup (Laryngotracheobronchitis)

- *CLASSIC PRESENTATION*: A child 3 months to 5 years of age with the insidious onset of fever, barking cough, inspiratory stridor, and mild respiratory distress.
- There is an increased incidence of croup in males.
- The peak incidence of croup is in the fall and winter.
- Most cases are caused by parainfluenza virus.
- Anterior-posterior (AP) neck x-ray may show the classic "steeple sign." Do an x-ray only if the child is not in significant respiratory distress!
- Treat with humidification and cool night air. If disease is severe enough to require hospitalization, oxygen with or without intubation, cool mist or croup tent, aerosolized racemic epinephrine, and corticosteroids can be used for treatment.

Epiglottitis

- *CLASSIC PRESENTATION*: The abrupt onset of high fever, moderate to severe respiratory distress, and stridor in a child who is sitting forward with his mouth open and drooling.
- Almost all cases are caused by *H. influenzae* type B.
- Epiglottitis is an emergency and the child should be admitted to the intensive care unit.
- Visualization of the epiglottis with a laryngoscope or bronchoscope in an operating room with full cardiorespiratory support is essential.
- The diagnosis is based on finding a swollen, cherry-red epiglottis.
- The thumbprint sign is seen on lateral x-ray (caused by enlarged epiglottis).
- Treat with intubation and ampicillin or a third generation cephalosporin.
- Do not give epinephrine or corticosteroids.

Whooping Cough

- *CLASSIC PRESENTATION*: A child with a two-week prodrome of upper respiratory infection followed by 2 weeks of paroxysmal, machine-gun-like cough and nasopharyngeal mucus that is strangling, thick, and clear. There is a stridorous inspiratory gasp at the end of each paroxysm ("whoop").
- The cough is often described as a staccato cough.
- This infection is caused by *Bordatella pertussis* but is rare due to immunization.
- Diagnose whooping cough by positive nasopharyngeal culture.
- Treat whooping cough with erythromycin.

Asthma

- *CLASSIC PRESENTATION*: A child with a history of intermittent wheezing with physical examination revealing wheezing, cough, chest pain, agitation, perioral cyanosis, intercostal and suprasternal retractions, and bilateral wheezing.
- Etiology is increased airway resistance due to bronchial mucosa edema, bronchospasm, and increased secretions.
- Asthma can be triggered by allergens, exercise, or cold weather.
- PO_2 is decreased due to poor oxygenation.
- PCO_2 is decreased initially due to hyperventilation.
- Chest x-ray often reveals hyperinflation with a flattened diaphragm.
- Treat with albuterol or inhaled steroids in cases of severe chronic asthma.

Foreign Body Aspiration

- *CLASSIC PRESENTATION*: A young child who suddenly begins choking and coughing while eating or playing with small objects. Physical examination reveals inspiratory stridor and mild intercostal and suprasternal retractions.
- If the victim can speak, breathe, or cough, interventions should be avoided.

- The foreign body most commonly lodges in the right mainstem bronchus.
- Chest x-ray may reveal hyper- or hypoinflation of the affected lung. The aspirated object may be seen if it is radiopaque.
- If intervention is required, back blows should be performed on children less than 1 year of age, and abdominal thrusts for children older than one year. In a controlled setting, the lodged object may be removed via rigid bronchoscopy.

GASTROINTESTINAL DISEASE

Pyloric Stenosis
- *CLASSIC PRESENTATION*: An infant 2 to 4 weeks old with projectile **nonbilious** vomiting, constipation, and poor weight gain. Physical examination reveals an olive-shaped abdominal mass with visible peristaltic waves traveling left to right across the abdomen.
- Males are more commonly affected, especially first-born males with a positive family history of pyloric stenosis.
- Treat with pyloromyotomy and correction of fluid and electrolyte abnormalities.

Duodenal Atresia
- *CLASSIC PRESENTATION*: A neonate with bilious vomiting within hours of first feeding and double-bubble sign on x-ray.
- Duodenal atresia is associated with Down's syndrome and prematurity.

Malrotation and Volvulus
- *CLASSIC PRESENTATION*: An infant who presents in the first year with bilious vomiting, intermittent abdominal pain, and crankiness. Physical examination may reveal a distended abdomen and evidence of dehydration.
- Malrotation and volvulus are caused by twisting of the bowel about the superior mesenteric artery with resulting obstruction and bilious vomiting.
- Eighty percent of sufferers present within the first 2 months of life.
- The infant may be shocky if the volvulus has progressed to bowel necrosis.
- Diagnose with an upper GI series.
- Emergent surgery is required.

Intussusception
- *CLASSIC PRESENTATION*: A child less than 2 years old with irritability, colicky abdominal pain, vomiting, rectal bleeding ("currant jelly stools"), and lethargy. Physical examination may reveal a sausage-like mass on abdominal examination.

- Intussusception is caused by invagination of one part of the intestine into another, commonly at the ileocecal valve. The most common "lead point" is a Meckel's diverticulum.
- Treat with IV hydration and antibiotics, followed by a diagnostic and often therapeutic air or barium enema.

Meckel's Diverticulum
- *CLASSIC PRESENTATION*: A child with painless rectal bleeding in the first 3 years of life.
- This is a remnant of the omphalomesenteric duct that contains pancreatic or gastric ectopic mucosa in 25% of cases.
- Remember the **rule of 2's**: 2% of the population, symptomatic 2% of the time, 2 feet from the ileocecal valve, 2:1 male:female ratio, and presentation before the age of 2.
- Intestinal obstruction pain that may mimic appendicitis can also be present.
- Treat Meckel's diverticulum with surgery.

Hirschsprung's Disease
- *CLASSIC PRESENTATION*: A neonate with failure to pass meconium within the first 24 hours of life followed by increasing difficulty with bowel movement leading to severe constipation.
- The absence of myenteric plexus innervation of the rectum or colon causes a functional obstruction.
- Males are more commonly affected by Hirschsprung's disease.
- A dilated proximal segment of colon can be seen on contrast enema.
- Megacolon may develop in the region proximal to the aganglionic segment.
- Hirschprung's disease is definitively diagnosed by the absence of myenteric ganglia on biopsy, but is often diagnosed with contrast enema.
- Treat with surgical resection of the aganglionic segment.

Crohn's Disease
- Crohn's disease can first be seen around age 10.
- It can be anywhere in the GI tract.
- Crohn's disease is associated with short stature, uveitis, and arthritis.
- Please see the Internal Medicine chapter for a full description of Crohn's disease.

Celiac Disease
- *CLASSIC PRESENTATION*: A child between 9 and 24 months (when new foods are being added to the diet) with vomiting, diarrhea, failure to thrive, abdominal distention, and irritability.

- Celiac disease is caused by an intolerance to gluten, which is present in barley, rye, oats, and wheat.
- Celiac disease is diagnosed with serologic screening for antibodies and small bowel biopsy that shows an absence of intestinal villi.

NEPHROLOGY

Nephrotic Syndrome
- *CLASSIC PRESENTATION*: A child between 2 to 5 years of age with proteinuria, hypoalbuminemia, edema, and hypercholesterolemia.
- Nephrotic syndrome is not a single disease; rather it may accompany any glomerular disease.
- Minimal change disease accounts for 80% of all cases of nephrotic syndrome in children.
- In addition to the above symptoms, fatigue, anorexia, abdominal pain, diarrhea, and intravascular volume depletion may be present.
- These patients have normal renal function, no hematuria, normal blood pressure, and normal serum complement levels.
- Minimal change disease is usually diagnosed by its response to steroid therapy.
- Minimal change disease usually follows a relapsing course, but most cases remit permanently by the end of adolescence. These patients are at increased risk of infection due to loss of complement.

Poststreptococcal Glomerulonephritis
- *CLASSIC PRESENTATION*: A child with hematuria, nephrotic syndrome, or renal failure about 10 days after having Strep throat or simply a sore throat.
- It is caused by Group A Streptococci.
- The glomerulonephritis is mediated by the inflammatory response to immune complex deposition.
- There will be decreased level of complement (C3).
- An antistreptolysin O (ASO) titer will usually be positive.
- RBC casts may be seen in the urine.

Urinary Tract Infection
- See Infectious Disease section

Pyelonephritis
- *CLASSIC PRESENTATION*: A patient who may have a history of urinary tract infection (UTI) symptoms presents with extreme flank tenderness, fever, vomiting, and an extremely ill appearance.
- The WBC is greater than 20,000 and the ESR is elevated.

- Flank tenderness may be difficult to elicit in infants.
- Children may also present with symptoms such as unexplained fever, failure to thrive, vague abdominal complaints, and bedwetting (enuresis).
- Pyelonephritis is most commonly caused by *E. coli*.
- Vesicoureteral reflux is present in one third of children with UTI.
- Imaging is indicated in the following cases:
  1. In all children younger than 2 years of age with a UTI.
  2. In all boys with a UTI.
  3. In all girls with pyelonephritis.
- Pyelonephritis may be treated with 10 to 14 days of oral antibiotic therapy.
- Ultrasonography should be performed to search for obstruction or congenital anomalies.
- Complications of UTI include hypertension and renal scarring.

Hypertension

- Hypertension is usually asymptomatic.
- A child with hypertension must always receive a thorough work-up to determine the etiology.
- The most common identifiable cause of hypertension in young children is renal in origin.
- Other common causes of hypertension include cystic disease, congenital vascular anomalies, tumor, and infection.

Nephritic Syndrome

- *CLASSIC PRESENTATION*: A child with hematuria, hypertension, and edema.
- Be sure to differentiate these symptoms from those of nephrotic syndrome.
- Alport's syndrome is a hereditary disorder, inherited as an X-linked or autosomal dominant trait, in which nephritis is associated with high-frequency sensorineural hearing loss.

NONCYANOTIC HEART DEFECTS

Atrial Septal Defect (ASD)

- Atrial septal defect is usually asymptomatic in childhood.
- Physical examination will reveal a wide or fixed split S2 heart sound, and there may also be a nonspecific systolic ejection murmur as a result of increased pulmonary flow.
- There is a left-to-right shunt at the atrial level, which, over time, may result in pulmonary hypertension and right ventricular hypertrophy.
- Treat with surgical closure of the defect.

Ventricular Septal Defect (VSD)

- VSD is the most common congenital heart disorder.
- Physical examination reveals a <u>harsh systolic murmur</u> that is loudest over the left sternal border.
- VSD eventually may lead to left ventricular hypertrophy.
- Large defects may lead to pulmonary hypertension and eventual reversal of flow across the defect.
- Bacterial endocarditis prophylaxis is indicated.
- A large VSD should be repaired before pulmonary vascular changes become irreversible.
- Small defects do not require surgical repair, and 50% of cases will close spontaneously.

Atrioventricular Septal Defects

- Atrioventricular septal defects are also known as endocardial cushion defects.
- Atrioventricular septal defects are most commonly associated with Down's syndrome.
- Diagnose with echocardiography.

Patent Ductus Arteriosus (PDA)

- PDA usually occurs as a result of prematurity.
- Physical examination reveals a continuous machine-like murmur that is loudest over the first and second intercostal spaces in the left midclavicular line.
- In a large shunt, bounding pulses may be palpated.
- A large PDA with a large left-to-right shunt may result in CHF, slowed growth, and repeated lower respiratory tract infections.
- The ductus arteriosus may be closed with indomethacin, but many require division and ligation or interventional catheterization.

Coarctation of the Aorta

- Coarctation of the aorta is associated with Turner's syndrome and bicuspid aortic valve.
- Blood pressures are higher in upper extremities than in lower extremities.
- The obstruction is usually located in the descending aorta.
- Chest x-ray may show the aortic knob and a dilated descending aorta, forming a "reverse 3" sign. Rib notching may also be seen.
- The treatment is surgical repair.

CYANOTIC HEART DEFECTS

The 5 T's (5 Cyanotic Heart Defects):
- Tetralogy of Fallot
- Tricuspid Atresia
- Truncus Arteriosus (persistent)
- Transposition of the Great Vessels
- Total Anomalous Pulmonary Venous Return

Tetralogy of Fallot
- *CLASSIC PRESENTATION*: A young child with cyanosis, squatting posture, hyperpnea, and dyspnea on exertion.
- This is the most common cyanotic congenital cardiac abnormality.
- The four defects are pulmonary stenosis, dextroposition of the aorta, ventricular septal defect, and right ventricular hypertrophy.
- A boot-shaped heart is the classic radiographic presentation.
- Hypoxemic (Tet) spells may be improved by placing the child in a knee-chest position.

Tricuspid Atresia
- Tricuspid atresia is often accompanied by a patent foramen ovale.
- A right-to-left atrial shunt is obligatory (VSD or patent ductus arteriosus).
- Prostaglandin E (PGE) may be used to maintain the patency of the ductus arteriosus.

Truncus Arteriosus
- This is a rare abnormality in which a single trunk exits from the heart.
- It is accompanied by a large VSD.
- This defect is surgically corrected by closing the VSD, incorporating the truncus in the left ventricle, and creating a conduit between the right ventricle and pulmonary arteries.

Transposition of the Great Vessels
- This is a defect in which the aorta arises from the right ventricle while the pulmonary artery arises from the left ventricle.
- Since unoxygenated blood is recirculated through the body, a lesion that allows mixing of the systemic and pulmonary circulations (ASD, VSD, PDA) is necessary for survival.
- It is surgically repaired by an arterial switch procedure.

Total Anomalous Pulmonary Venous Return

- In this defect, the pulmonary veins carry oxygenated blood to the right atrium rather than the left.
- There is an obligatory right-to-left shunt, usually a foramen ovale or PDA.
- This defect is surgically repaired by connecting the pulmonary veins to the left atrium.

HEMATOLOGY

Iron Deficiency Anemia

- *CLASSIC PRESENTATION*: A child between 6 and 24 months who is on a diet consisting almost entirely of milk and who is irritable, anorexic, lethargic, and easily fatiguable.
- Iron deficiency is the most common cause of anemia in children.
- Microcytic hypochromic RBCs are seen on smear.
- Common laboratory findings include decreased hemoglobin, serum iron levels, and serum ferritin.
- Increased total iron binding capacity and erythrocyte protoporphyrin are also seen.
- Treat with elemental iron for 2 to 3 months after the hemoglobin level has returned to normal. If there is no response to iron therapy, consider other causes for the anemia.

Sickle Cell Anemia

- *CLASSIC PRESENTATION*: Sickle cell anemia is the most common cause of hemolytic anemia in the African-American population.
- About 10% of African Americans are heterozygous (carriers) for the Hb S gene.
- Sickle cell anemia is caused by the substitution of valine for glutamic acid in the sixth position of the β-chain of hemoglobin.
- Autosplenectomy is common and usually the spleen is no longer palpable by 5 years.
- Note that children with sickle cell anemia do not respond to pneumococcal vaccine until about 2 years of age.
- Hypoxia, dehydration, chilling, infection, and acidosis can cause sickling of RBCs, resulting in vaso-occlusive episodes.
- Vaso-occlusive episodes can produce pain in the abdomen, bones, or chest, as well as cerebrovascular accident and pulmonary infarction.
- Howell-Jolly bodies are seen on peripheral smear.
- Sickle cell anemia patients are at increased risk of overwhelming infection, and therefore should be immunized against *H. influenzae*, *Pneumococcus*, and *Meningococcus*.
- Daily oral penicillin should be given prophylactically.
- Parents should be taught to treat febrile illnesses as potential sepsis.

Hemophilia A (Factor VIII Deficiency)

- *CLASSIC PRESENTATION*: A male with history of easy bruising that often becomes more frequent when he is old enough to walk. The child may have a history of neonatal bleeding, especially with circumcision.
- Due to factor VIII procoagulant defect (VIII:C).
- Hemophilia A is more common than Hemophilia B.
- There is X-linked recessive inheritance, usually with a positive family history.
- PTT is prolonged, decreased factor VIII level.
- Clinical manifestations include soft tissue bleeding and painful hemarthrosis of the ankles, knees, and elbows.
- Treat with factor VIII replacement.

Von Willebrand's Disease

- *CLASSIC PRESENTATION*: A child who presents with a history of easy bruising and bleeding with or without trauma.
- Von Willebrand's disease is the most common inherited bleeding disorder.
- Most often there is an undetectable level of von Willebrand factor and decreased level of factor VIII due to decreased production of factor VIII. This results in the inability of platelets to adhere to damaged endothelium.
- Disease severity varies with the degree of deficiency. Usually there is only mucosal and cutaneous bleeding.
- There is prolonged bleeding time and prolonged PTT.
- Treat with DDAVP, cryoprecipitate, or factor VIII concentrates.

Hemophilia B (Christmas disease)

- Clinical features are similar to hemophilia A.
- Hemophilia B is due to factor IX deficiency.
- Hemophilia B is an X-linked recessive disorder.
- PTT is prolonged.

Thalassemia

- *CLASSIC PRESENTATION*: An infant or older child with easy bruising and/or bleeding.
- Thalassemia is due to decreased synthesis of globin chains.
- α-thalassemia is more common in Asian and African populations.
- β-thalassemia is more common in Mediterranean and African population.

ONCOLOGY

Common Types of Childhood Cancer
- Leukemia and solid tumors represent the majority of childhood neoplasms.
- Acute lymphoblastic leukemia (ALL) is the most common pediatric neoplasm.

Leukemias
- *CLASSIC PRESENTATION*: A child may present with one or many of the following signs and symptoms: fatigue, fever, pallor, petechiae, purpura, weight loss, anorexia, lymphadenopathy, bone or joint pain, hepatosplenomegaly.
- Acute leukemias represent 95% of all childhood leukemias.
- Acute lymphoblastic leukemia (ALL) is the most common type of childhood leukemia (75% of all leukemias).
- ALL is most common between 3 to 5 years.
- The clinical features of leukemias are often similar to those of aplastic anemia.
- Anemia may result in pallor, irritability, and decreased activity.
- Superficial bleeding occurs due to thrombocytopenia.
- Infection occurs due to leukopenia.
- The CNS and testes act as sanctuary sites and are important as sites of recurrence.
- Treat with chemotherapy and CNS irradiation.

Non-Hodgkin's Lymphoma (NHL)
- *CLASSIC PRESENTATION*: An adolescent presents with an anterior mediastinal mass, abdominal mass, or peripheral lymph node enlargement.
- NHL is seen most commonly in older children, teenagers, and males.
- Treated with extensive surgical debulking, systemic chemotherapy, and CNS prophylaxis.

Hodgkin's Disease
- *CLASSIC PRESENTATION*: An adolescent who presents with localized adenopathy, fever, night sweats, and weight loss.
- Hodgkin's disease occurs in older children, teenagers. It has a slight female predominance.
- In Hodgkin's disease, look for supraclavicular and cervical lymph node involvement.
- Reed-Sternberg cells are pathognomonic.
- Treat Hodgkin's disease with radiotherapy and sometimes chemotherapy.

Most Common Solid Tumors in Order of Frequency

- Brain tumors (medulloblastoma and astrocytoma)
- Wilms' tumor
- Neuroblastoma
- Soft tissue sarcoma

Brain Tumors

- Most occur below the tentorium.
- Astrocytoma arises primarily above the tentorium and presents with focal neurologic deficits, signs of increased intracranial pressure, and focal seizures.
- Medulloblastoma characteristically presents as a cerebellar tumor resulting in signs of increased intracranial pressure and cerebellar signs.

Wilms' Tumor

- *CLASSIC PRESENTATION*: A 2-year-old child presents with a large, painless abdominal mass. The child may have hypertension.
- Wilms' tumor usually occurs in first 5 years of life.
- This is an embryonal tumor of renal origin.
- It is associated with hemihypertrophy, aniridia, GU abnormalities, and mental retardation.
- Treat Wilms' tumor with surgery, radiotherapy, and chemotherapy.

Neuroblastoma

- *CLASSIC PRESENTATION*: A child less than 2 years old who presents with a painless abdominal mass. The child may also present with abdominal pain and/or hypertension if the mass is displacing the kidneys.
- Neuroblastoma is a malignancy of neural crest cells of the paraspinal sympathetic ganglia and adrenal medulla.
- Head and neck tumors can result in Horner's syndrome.
- Urinary tumor markers include vanillylmandelic acid and homovanillic acid.
- Treat neuroblastoma with surgery and sometimes chemotherapy.
- Infants younger than 1 year of age have the best prognosis.

Rhabdomyosarcoma

- Rhabdomyosarcoma may occur in the orbit, nasopharynx, middle ear, neck, GU tract, or extremities.
- These are tumors that arise from mesenchyme and have characteristics of skeletal muscle.

Ewing's Sarcoma

- *CLASSIC PRESENTATION*: An adolescent male with hip pain followed by swelling.
- Ewing's sarcoma is primarily seen in adolescents and is more common in males.
- Common sites of Ewing's sarcoma are the proximal femur and pelvic bones.
- An x-ray classically reveals an "onion skin" appearance of the bone as a result of disruption of the cortex with layers of new periosteal bone formation.
- Radiotherapy is the main form of treatment. For aggressive tumors, radiotherapy and chemotherapy may be used before surgical excision.

Osteogenic Sarcoma

- *CLASSIC PRESENTATION*: A boy who presents with persistent knee pain after minor knee trauma. There may be a palpable mass on physical examination.
- Osteogenic sarcoma is the most common primary malignant bone tumor seen in children, with an increased incidence in males.
- Most cases of osteogenic sarcoma occur near the knee joint (distal femur, proximal tibia).
- X-ray classically reveals periosteal elevation with a "sunburst" pattern of soft-tissue calcification.
- This tumor most commonly metastasizes to the lungs.
- Alkaline phosphatase is a tumor marker.

VASCULITIDES

Henoch-Schönlein Purpura

- *CLASSIC PRESENTATION*: A young child who presents with petechiae or palpable purpura over the buttocks and lower extremities, which is associated with abdominal pain, arthritis, or glomerulonephritis.
- A normal platelet count and coagulation studies differentiate Henoch-Schönlein purpura from other hemorrhagic disorders.
- This is the most common vasculitis of childhood.
- The purpura is a vasculitis that results from the deposition of IgA immune complexes.
- Fifty percent of patients also have nephritis.
- The disease has a self-limited course of 4 to 6 weeks, and treatment is symptomatic.

Idiopathic Thrombocytopenic Purpura (ITP)

- *CLASSIC PRESENTATION*: A child who presents with the abrupt onset of bleeding of the skin and mucous membranes following a viral illness or immunization. The platelet count is low, which helps to differentiate it from Henoch-Schönlein purpura.

- Most cases resolve spontaneously in 1 to 6 months.
- Treatment is conservative unless the platelet count drops below 10,000.
- ITP can be treated with steroids or intravenous gamma globulin.

Kawasaki's Disease (Mucocutaneous Lymph Node Syndrome)
- *CLASSIC PRESENTATION*: An Asian child younger than 4 years of age with the following symptoms:
- In order to make the diagnosis, the child must have had a fever for at least 5 days and have four out of the five "RULES":
  > *R*ash
  > *U*nilateral lymphadenopathy in cervical region
  > *L*ip/oral findings (red cracked lips, strawberry tongue)
  > *E*xtremity findings (edema, induration, or desquamation)
  > *S*ymmetric conjunctivitis
- The etiology of Kawasaki's disease is unknown, but an infection may lead to an immune-mediated disease in genetically predisposed persons.
- The major complication of this disease is the development of coronary artery aneurysms.
- Intravenous gamma globulin given early in the course of the illness can decrease the risk of coronary artery aneurysm.
- High doses of aspirin are given during the acute phase for the anti-inflammatory effect.
- After the child is afebrile, low doses of aspirin are given for the antithrombotic effect.

CHROMOSOMAL DISORDERS

Trisomy 21 (Down's Syndrome)
- *CLASSIC PRESENTATION*: A child with flat facies, upslanting palpebral fissures, flat nasal bridge with epicanthal folds, protruding tongue, short stature and a single transverse palmar crease. Infants may present with hypotonia, flattened occiput, redundant skin on the posterior neck, and small ears.
- An analysis of karyotype shows an extra chromosome 21 in about 90% of all cases.
- The risk of having a child with Down's syndrome (and other aneuploid syndromes) increases with advancing maternal age.
- Fifty percent have congenital heart disease, the most common being endocardial cushion defects (defects of the A-V canal).
- Duodenal atresia is common. This is classically seen as a double-bubble sign on abdominal radiograph.

- Hypothyroidism and leukemia occur at a higher frequency in persons with Down's syndrome.
- Many experience a dementia in the third or fourth decade of life which resembles Alzheimer's disease.

Trisomy 13 (Patau's Syndrome)

- *CLASSIC PRESENTATION*: A child with severe birth defects including microcephaly, cleft lip/palate, holoprosencephaly, polydactyly, severe mental retardation, congenital heart disease, and omphalocele.
- Most children die in the first year of life, and survivors are usually severely mentally retarded.

Trisomy 18 (Edwards' Syndrome)

- Most cases are due to nondisjunction.
- Trisomy 18 is associated with intrauterine growth retardation, microcephaly, severe mental retardation, hypertonia, and a small mandible.
- Most patients die before 1 year of age, and survivors are usually retarded.

AUTOSOMAL DOMINANT DISORDERS

General

- Recurrence risk is 50% for an individual with an autosomal dominant disorder.
- There may be variable expressivity with varying degrees of severity among affected individuals.
- Examples of autosomal dominant disorders are Huntington's disease, neurofibromatosis, tuberous sclerosis, and Marfan's syndrome.

Marfan's Syndrome

- *CLASSIC PRESENTATION*: A disproportionately tall individual with long, thin face, extremities, and digits, hypermobile joints, and possibly scoliosis.
- Marfan's syndrome is caused by abnormal fibrillin that results in connective tissue abnormalities.
- Cardiac abnormalities include aortic root dilatation, mitral valve prolapse, and aneurysms.
- Ophthalmologic features include severe myopia and lens subluxation.
- Pulmonary complications include spontaneous pneumothorax and emphysema.
- β-blockers may be effective in reducing progression to aortic root dilatation.

AUTOSOMAL RECESSIVE DISORDERS

General
- Recurrence risk is 25% for two carrier parents to have a child with an autosomal recessive disorder.
- Examples of autosomal recessive disorders are sickle cell disease and cystic fibrosis.

Cystic Fibrosis
- *CLASSIC PRESENTATION*: A Caucasian child with a history of meconium ileus at birth who presents with chronic diarrhea and recurrent pneumonias. Parents may complain that the baby has a "salty taste."
- Cystic fibrosis is the most common autosomal recessive disorder in whites of European descent.
- Cystic fibrosis is due to a defect in membrane transport of chloride, most often the delta-F508 mutation.
- Cystic fibrosis is diagnosed with the sweat chloride test, which reveals excessive levels of chloride in the sweat.
- Intestinal malabsorption is due to decreased pancreatic exocrine function.

SEX CHROMOSOME DISORDERS

Turner's Syndrome
- *CLASSIC PRESENTATION*: A short female with webbing of the neck, a shield-shaped chest, low posterior hairline, and multiple pigmented nevi.
- In this defect, only one X chromosome exists or is normal.
- All patients have gonadal dysgenesis (primary amenorrhea).
- Fifty percent of patients have kidney malformations.
- Turner's syndrome is associated with coarctation of the aorta and a bicuspid aortic valve.
- Intelligence is normal but some spatial perceptual difficulties have been noted.

Klinefelter's Syndrome
- *CLASSIC PRESENTATION*: A male with 47, XXY karyotype.
- Clinical features include tall stature, incomplete masculinization with gynecoid pelvis, gynecomastia, small testes (often undescended), and behavioral problems.

X-LINKED DISORDERS

Fragile X Syndrome
- *CLASSIC PRESENTATION*: A male infant with mental retardation, macro-orchidism, and characteristic facial features including a long face, prominent forehead, long chin, and large prominent ears.
- Fragile X syndrome is diagnosed by growing the patient's cells in a medium with a low folic acid concentration.

Duchenne's Muscular Dystrophy
- *CLASSIC PRESENTATION*: A male child about 3 years old with a waddling gait and difficulty climbing stairs who is found to have enlarged calf muscles upon physical examination.
- Duchenne's muscular dystrophy is caused by a lack of **dystrophin** in the muscle membrane.
- This is an X-linked recessive disorder.
- The serum creatine phosphokinase level is 10 to 20 times normal.
- There is progressive muscle weakness seen first in the proximal muscles.
- Patients are usually wheelchair-bound by 12 years of age and die young.

INBORN ERRORS OF METABOLISM

Phenylketonuria (PKU)
- *CLASSIC PRESENTATION*: A child who is asymptomatic early in infancy but later develops mental retardation, hypopigmentation, hypertonicity, and behavioral disorders.
- PKU is due to deficiency in the enzyme phenylalanine hydroxylase.
- If left untreated, an individual with PKU will be hypopigmented (often a very pale-skinned African American), mentally retarded, and neurologically impaired with hypertonicity, tremors, or behavior disorders.
- Newborn screening programs exist in most states.
- Treatment includes dietary restriction of phenylalanine intake to prevent symptoms.

POISONING AND CHILD ABUSE

Acetaminophen
- There are 4 phases of acetaminophen overdose:
  Phase I (begins about one hour after ingestion and lasts up to 24 hours)
  Most patients do not progress beyond this stage

GI signs such as anorexia, nausea, vomiting, and diaphoresis
Phase II (24-48 hours)
  Resolution of GI symptoms
  Abdominal tenderness
  Elevated LFTs and bilirubin
Phase III (3-4 days)
  Anorexia, nausea, vomiting, malaise
  LFTs peak
Phase IV (4 days-2 weeks)
  Resolution of symptoms and liver abnormalities if the patient
  survives the first 3 phases.

- Acetaminophen ingestion is treated with N-acetylcysteine.

Child Abuse Risk Factors

- Poverty
- Social isolation of the caregiver
- Marital disharmony
- Financial difficulties in the family
- Parental alcoholism
- Young parents
- Prematurity of the infant
- If sexual abuse is suspected, cultures of the mouth, vagina, rectum and urethra should be obtained.

NOTES

Chapter 2

OBSTETRICS

Susan L. Taylor, M.D.

PREGNANCY

General

- Pregnancy should be considered in any female patient of reproductive age with amenorrhea, especially when prescribing any medications. Pregnancy can present as nausea, vomiting, fatigue, breast tenderness, pedal edema, urinary frequency, abdominal pain, amenorrhea, or a change in vaginal bleeding or discharge.
- Standard laboratory urine human chorionic gonadotropin (β-hCG) tests become positive approximately 4 weeks after the first day of the last menstrual period. Serum pregnancy tests are more sensitive and specific and can allow detection even before the patient misses a period.
- The most reliable indicators of pregnancy are detection of fetal heartbeat, ultrasonographic detection of a gestational sac, and recognition of fetal movements. Fetal heart rate by Doppler echocardiography should be present by 12 weeks. Initial maternal perception of fetal movement (quickening) usually occurs by 19 to 20 weeks. Chadwick's sign (congestion and a bluish discoloration of the cervix and vagina) and Hegar's sign (softening of the lower uterine segment) are also found early in pregnancy.
- To denote obstetrical history, use G#P#. G means gravida, and stands for the number of pregnancies (complete or incomplete) that the patient has ever had. P means para, and stands for the number of births that the patient has produced. Thus a G2P1 patient has been pregnant twice and given birth once.
- Abortion is defined as delivery of a fetus of 500 gm or less or delivery before 20 weeks. Premature delivery is defined as delivery between weeks 20 and 37. Postterm delivery is defined as delivery after 42 weeks gestation.

Prenatal Care

- All women who are pregnant or planning to become pregnant should be consuming 0.4 mg/day of folic acid to reduce their risk of having a fetus afflicted with neural tube defects. Most women should also be taking iron during pregnancy to help prevent iron deficiency anemia during pregnancy.
- Normal pregnancy lasts 40 plus or minus 2 weeks, calculated from the first day of the last normal menses (gestational age). Calculation of the due date is accomplished by adding 7 days to the first day of the last normal menstrual flow and counting back 3 months.
- Ultrasonic examination is the most accurate method for determining gestational age. In the first trimester (8 to 12 weeks), transvaginal ultrasound allows determination of gestational age to within 1 week. In the second trimester, accuracy is still high, in the 2-week range. In the third trimester, accuracy decreases to 3 weeks.

- For a patient with a normal pregnancy, periodic antepartum visits at 4-week intervals are usually scheduled until 32 weeks, then at 2-week intervals until 36 weeks, then weekly thereafter until delivery.
- The only routine laboratory test performed at every prenatal visit is determination of glucose and protein in urine.

Teratogens

Known Teratogens	Effects
phenytoin	mild mental retardation, growth retardation, facial anomalies, cardiac defects
warfarin	nasal hypoplasia, epiphyseal stippling, optic atrophy, mental retardation
alcohol	Fetal Alcohol Syndrome: growth retardation, mild mental retardation, midfacial hypoplasia, cardiac (especially ventricular septal) defects
methotrexate	abortion, multiple malformations
diethylstilbestrol (DES)	vaginal adenosis and clear cell carcinoma, cervical and uterine anomalies
thalidomide	congenital absence of arms, legs, hands, or feet (phocomelia)
valproic acid	open neural tube defects
isotretinoin	microtia, micrognathia, cardiovascular anomalies, neural tube defects

Smoking

- Smoking is associated with decreased fertility, increased placental abruption, increased perinatal mortality, ovulatory and tubal disorders, bleeding complications of pregnancy, decreased mean birth weight, small-for-gestational age babies, and preterm deliveries.
- Fetal hemoglobin has a higher affinity for carbon monoxide than does adult hemoglobin. This results in decreased fetal oxygen supply.
- Nicotine causes the adrenal gland to release increased amounts of epinephrine, norepinephrine, and acetylcholine, which leads to a decrease in uteroplacental perfusion.

FETAL EVALUATION

General
- Birth defects have a 2 to 4% incidence in the general population.

α-Fetoprotein
- Maternal serum α-fetoprotein (MSAFP) is normally measured during weeks 15 to 18.
- Elevated values are associated with increased risk of open neural tube defects (NTDs). A normal value rules out open NTDs with an 80 to 90% probability.
- Other causes of increased MSAFP include advanced gestational age, twins, threatened abortion, fetal death, maternal hepatitis, and Rh disease.
- A decreased MSAFP indicates an increased risk for Down's syndrome. When MSAFP is decreased, a triple marker assay should be performed (MSAFP, unconjugated estriol, and serum hCG).
- Women with low MSAFP, low unconjugated estriol, and increased serum hCG are more likely to have a Down's syndrome fetus.

Amniocentesis
- Amniocentesis is the transabdominal aspiration of fluid from the amniotic sac. Biochemical studies can identify the presence of fetal physiologic markers or substances indicating fetal abnormalities, such as α-fetoprotein in NTDs or bilirubin in Rh incompatibility.
- Amniocentesis can be performed after 15 weeks. It is associated with a 0.5% risk of fetal loss.
- Tissue culture of fetal cells allows genetic evaluation of the fetus.
- In more advanced gestations, amniocentesis can be used to assess the degree of fetal lung maturity by surfactant assays. Lecithin/sphingomyelin (L/S) ratio of less than 2 indicates poor fetal lung maturation and an increased risk of respiratory distress in the newborn. Identification of phosphatidylglycerol by amniocentesis is also an indicator of fetal lung maturity.

Chorionic Villus Sampling
- Chorionic villus sampling (CVS) is the aspiration of chorionic villi for genetic analysis of an early gestation.
- CVS can be performed earlier than amniocentesis (at 9 to 12 weeks), allowing for earlier detection of anomalies.
- Because CVS carries at least a 0.5% risk of fetal loss, it is usually reserved for patients with a greater risk of genetic abnormalities, such as women over 35 or with a history of genetic abnormalities.

Assessment of Fetal Well-being

- Fetal kick counts are a reliable, inexpensive, and commonly used test of fetal well-being.
- The nonstress test (NST) measures the response of the fetal heart rate to fetal movement.
- A normal, or reactive, nonstress test occurs when the fetal heart rate increases by at least 15 beats per minute over a period of 15 seconds following a fetal movement. Two such accelerations in a 20-minute span is considered normal.
- A nonreactive NST must be immediately followed with further assessment of fetal well-being, often by a biophysical profile.

Contraction Stress Test

- The contraction stress test (CST) measures the response of the fetal heart rate to uterine contractions, using either oxytocin infusion or nipple stimulation.
- During contractions, uteroplacental blood flow is temporarily reduced. A healthy fetus is able to compensate for this without changes in the basal heart rate or decelerations. However, a compromised fetus is unable to do so.
- If late decelerations are present, the test is considered positive, and delivery of the baby is indicated.

Ultrasonography

- Ultrasonography is used to assess amniotic fluid volume, fetal breathing, fetal tone, and fetal movement.
- A biophysical profile combines these four ultrasound assessments with a nonstress test to predict perinatal outcome.

MEDICAL DISORDERS DURING PREGNANCY

Gestational Diabetes Mellitus (GDM)

- *CLASSIC PRESENTATION:* A pregnant female, usually asymptomatic, with a family history of Type II diabetes mellitus, previous pregnancy with GDM, or any risk factor for Type II diabetes mellitus. She is found to have an elevated blood glucose on routine screening or after a 1-hour glucose tolerance test.
- A woman is more likely to develop glucose intolerance during pregnancy because of counterinsulin hormones and enzymes produced primarily by the placenta.
- Approximately 5% of American women will have documented glucose intolerance during pregnancy.
- GDM increases risk of fetal loss, fetal macrosomia and its complications (increased risk of operative or mechanical deliveries), and later development of Type II diabetes mellitus.

- Screening for GDM is routine at 24 to 28 weeks gestation, usually with a 1-hour glucose tolerance (Glucola) test. Screening should be done earlier in the presence of risk factors.
- Treatment is via tight control of blood glucose, using the same options as for other diabetics. These options include diet, oral hypoglycemics, and insulin. Treatment lowers the risk for most of the above complications.

Type I Diabetes Mellitus

- Tight control of blood glucose during pregnancy is mandatory ASAP (before conception if possible). This will lower the risk for most complications.
- Maternal complications of Type I diabetes mellitus include polyhydramnios and preeclampsia.
- Fetal complications include macrosomia and birth defects.

Chronic Hypertension

- *CLASSIC PRESENTATION:* A woman with a history of hypertension with sustained elevation of the blood pressure (> 140/90 mm Hg) before pregnancy or before the 20th week.
- Methyldopa is the drug of choice for antepartum treatment because it poses minimal risk to the fetus. Other medicines often used include β_1-blockers and nifedipine.
- Hospitalization is indicated for persistent elevation of blood pressure with values 30/15 mm Hg above previous levels, or if there are signs of preeclampsia or fetal compromise.
- Consider delivery when fetal lung maturity is attained, or by 40 weeks if fetal growth has been normal and maternal blood pressure well controlled.

Preeclampsia/Eclampsia

- *CLASSIC PRESENTATION:* A young woman with her first pregnancy who is found to have a large uterus for her dates (note that large babies, multiple gestations, polyhydramnios, and molar pregnancy are all risk factors). On physical examination after 20 weeks, her blood pressure is noted to be elevated >140/90 mm Hg or >30/15 mm Hg above baseline levels obtained before 20 weeks.
- Pregnancy-induced hypertension is more common than chronic hypertension during pregnancy. It affects up to 10% of all pregnancies.
- Preeclampsia is defined as hypertension, proteinuria, and edema of the hands and face.
- Eclampsia is defined as preeclampsia plus grand mal seizures. The seizures can occur before, during, and after delivery.
- HELLP Syndrome is associated with preeclampsia or eclampsia and consists of **H**emolytic anemia, **E**levated **L**iver enzymes, and **L**ow **P**latelets.

- Disorders of pregnancy-induced hypertension should be treated with bedrest, hypertensive medications if needed (hydralazine, β-blockers), and delivery when appropriate fetal lung maturity is attained.
- Treat or prevent seizures with magnesium sulfate.
- After delivery, observe closely and continue magnesium sulfate for at least 24 hours.

Thromboembolic Disease

- *CLASSIC PRESENTATION:* A pregnant woman, or a woman who has just delivered a baby, who complains of either calf pain or the sudden onset of shortness of breath and pleuritic chest pain.
- Patients at high risk for thromboembolic disease include those with advanced maternal age, high parity, obesity, immobility, diabetes mellitus, hypertension, cardiac disease, or severe varicose veins.
- During the antepartum period, the prevalence of deep venous thrombosis (DVT) remains similar to that found in nonpregnant women, but it increases four-fold to six-fold during labor, delivery, and the postpartum period.
- Women who have experienced a thromboembolic event before pregnancy have a 12% risk of recurrence.
- Diagnosis is the same as for nonpregnant patients and includes duplex studies of leg veins, a V/Q scan, and angiography.
- Treatment with IV heparin decreases the probability of pulmonary embolism and decreases overall mortality. (Remember, warfarin is a teratogen!)

Drug Abuse

- Cocaine use leads to increased risk of placental abruption, spontaneous abortion, growth retardation, stillbirth, and malformation. Affected infants usually have depressed interactive behavior and poor response to stimuli.
- Amphetamines have been shown to cause symmetrical fetal growth retardation.
- Alcohol use causes fetal alcohol syndrome.
- Opiate use leads to intrauterine withdrawal with increased fetal activity, neonatal withdrawal, increased rates of intrauterine growth retardation and intrauterine fetal demise. Give methadone maintenance therapy to mothers using opiates to prevent neonatal withdrawal.

Seizure Disorders

- Seizure disorders occur in 1% of pregnant women. The risk of a seizure disorder worsening during pregnancy is 50%. However, the risk is greater with recent seizures.
- Ideally, seizures should be prevented during pregnancy. However, remember that all anticonvulsants are teratogens.

- During pregnancy, try to use only one anticonvulsant medication, and select an effective one with the lowest teratogenic potential.
- Measure drug levels frequently during pregnancy. Consider discontinuing anticonvulsants if the patient has been seizure-free for at least 2 years.
- Patients should be given folic acid and vitamin K supplements (anticonvulsants often cause vitamin K deficiency in newborns).
- Status epilepticus should be treated vigorously. Once an airway is ensured, give IV diazepam, followed by IV phenytoin when serum drug levels are back.
- During labor, give magnesium sulfate or phenytoin for seizure prophylaxis.

Hyperthyroidism
- Hyperthyroidism is the most common endocrine disorder of pregnancy.
- Hyperthyroidism increases the risk of premature delivery and stillbirth.
- Remember, an elevated T_3/T_4 level is normal in pregnancy as a result of an increase in the level of thyroid binding globulin (TBG). However, the free (unbound) thyroid hormone levels and TSH should be normal.
- Treatment is with propylthiouracil.

ANTEPARTUM OBSTETRIC COMPLICATIONS

First Trimester Bleeding
- Causes of first trimester bleeding include incorrect menstrual dating, threatened or incomplete abortion, lesions of the cervix, ectopic pregnancy, missed abortion, and trophoblastic disease.
- First trimester bleeding should be considered a threatened abortion until another more specific diagnosis can be made.
- Serum quantitative hCG testing will identify abnormal pregnancies, ectopic pregnancy, or those destined to abort in most cases if a rate of increase of less than 66% over 48 hours is noted.
- Pelvic ultrasound is used to confirm the presence of an intrauterine pregnancy and/or to look for an ectopic pregnancy.

Spontaneous Abortion
- Spontaneous abortion is defined as spontaneous termination of a pregnancy prior to fetal viability, usually defined as less than 20 weeks or less than 500 g.
- Some authorities believe that up to 80% of all conceptions fail to produce viable offspring. Many pregnancies fail early on, even before pregnancy is detected.
- Risk factors for spontaneous abortion include high parity, increasing maternal age, increasing paternal age, previous spontaneous abortions, and conception within 3 months of a live birth.

- The most common cause of spontaneous abortion is chromosomal or genetic abnormalities of the fetus.
- Other etiologies of spontaneous abortion include uterine abnormalities, endocrine abnormalities (diabetes mellitus and hyperthyroidism), immunologic dysfunction, infection, smoking, alcohol, toxins, and radiation.
- A threatened abortion is defined as uterine bleeding without cervical dilation or effacement. About 50% of threatened abortions will abort. Treat with bedrest and pelvic rest.
- An inevitable abortion is defined as uterine bleeding with cervical dilation but without passage of tissues. Treat by awaiting spontaneous passage or by surgical completion (dilation and curettage).
- An incomplete abortion is defined as cervical dilation with profuse bleeding and partial passage of tissue. Treat with surgical completion of the abortion.
- A complete abortion is defined as cervical dilation and complete passage of tissue, usually with minimal bleeding and cramps. No treatment is necessary.
- A missed abortion is defined as intrauterine fetal death without tissue passage for more than 8 weeks. The mother is at risk of disseminated intravascular coagulation (DIC) secondary to release of fetal tissue thromboplastin. The risk increases with increasing time since fetal death. Treatment is surgical completion of the abortion.
- A septic abortion is defined as an abortion caused by or complicated by infection. One to 2% of spontaneous abortions are septic. Treatment is surgical completion and IV antibiotics.
- If the mother is Rh-negative, always give Rh immune globulin after spontaneous abortion or any time that maternal blood may come in contact with fetal blood.

Ectopic Pregnancy
- *CLASSIC PRESENTATION:* A woman of reproductive age or known pregnancy in the first trimester who presents with amenorrhea, abnormal vaginal bleeding, and abdominal pain. A pregnancy test is positive and an ultrasound reveals the absence of intrauterine pregnancy.
- Risk factors for ectopic pregnancy include prior ectopic pregnancy (ten-fold increased risk), history of PID/salpingitis, tubal ligation, and IUD use.
- Most ectopic pregnancies occur in the uterine tube (95%). Other uncommon locations include the cervix, ovary, and peritoneum.
- Rupture of an ectopic pregnancy is an acute emergency and can cause the mother to bleed to death. Only about 5% of women with ruptured ectopic pregnancies present in hypovolemic shock initially.
- Diagnosis: Serial quantitative levels of β-hCG can be followed at 2-day intervals. Early in pregnancy, β-hCG levels should increase by at least 66% in 48 hours. A smaller increase indicates a pregnancy not growing appropriately, thus increasing the suspicion of ectopic pregnancy. A useful adjunct to quantitative β-hCG is ultrasound.

- Transabdominal ultrasound should identify intrauterine gestation by the time the β-hCG is 5000-6000 IU/L, and transvaginal ultrasound by the time the β-hCG is 1500 IU/L. The most accurate diagnosis is by direct visualization with laparoscopy or laparotomy.
- Treatment traditionally consists of surgical removal of the fetus. However, selected small unruptured ectopics can be treated with methotrexate or expectant management (hoping for spontaneous regression).
- Rh-negative mothers with ectopics should receive Rh immune globulin to prevent Rh sensitization.

Rh Isoimmunization/Hemolytic Disease of the Newborn

- Isoimmunization is the development of antibodies to red blood cell antigens following exposure to such antigens from another individual (such as a fetus). The Rh system is most commonly involved in isoimmunization, and the antigen most commonly associated with hemolytic disease of the newborn is the D antigen.
- When a fetus is Rh-positive (has inherited the D antigen from its father), and the mother is Rh-negative (has no D antigen), the conditions exist for isoimmunization.
- At delivery, if the mother's blood is exposed to fetal RBCs the mother can develop antibodies to the D antigen. In a subsequent pregnancy, the mother can pass IgG antibodies across the placenta, which will lead to hemolytic anemia in the fetus.
- In severe cases, this can lead to high output cardiac failure in the fetus and hydrops fetalis.
- As part of routine antenatal laboratory evaluation, maternal blood is tested for the Rh status as well as for the presence of other common antibodies which can cause disturbances in the newborn.
- Rh-negative patients who have no antibody on initial screen are retested at 28 weeks. If no sensitization has occurred, patients are given Rh immune globulin (RhoGAM) to protect them for the remainder of pregnancy.
- Administration of Rh immune globulin soon after delivery can, by passive immunization, prevent an active antibody response by the mother, in most cases. It is now standard of care for all Rh-negative mothers to receive Rh immune globulin within 72 hours of delivery.
- Indications for Rh immune globulin in an unsensitized Rh-negative patient include:
    1. A pregnancy at 28 weeks
    2. Delivery of an Rh-positive infant within the last 72 hours
    3. At the time of amniocentesis
    4. After a positive Betke-Kleihauer test (for fetal RBCs in maternal circulation)
    5. After an ectopic pregnancy
    6. After a spontaneous or induced abortion

7.   Any other circumstance in pregnancy in which fetomaternal hemorrhage can occur

Preterm Labor

- *CLASSIC PRESENTATION:* A pregnant woman who presents between 20 and 36 weeks gestation with regular uterine contractions, occurring with a frequency of 10 minutes or less, and each contraction lasting at least 30 seconds. Physical examination reveals cervical effacement, dilation, and/or descent of the fetus into the pelvis.
- Factors associated with preterm labor include dehydration, infection (particularly UTI), premature rupture of membranes (PROM), incompetent cervix, excessive uterine enlargement or distortion, placental abnormalities, maternal smoking, and substance abuse.
- Preterm labor and delivery are associated with neonatal complications such as respiratory distress syndrome (RDS), intraventricular hemorrhage, neonatal infection, necrotizing enterocolitis, and sepsis.
- Treatment for preterm labor includes pelvic rest, hydration, and detection and treatment of any disorders associated with preterm labor.
- If labor continues, tocolytics can be used, including magnesium sulfate, β_2-agonists (terbutaline and ritodrine), prostaglandin synthetase inhibitors (indomethacin), and calcium channel blockers (nifedipine).
- Relatively early in the third trimester (28 to 32 weeks), management should include administration of glucocorticoid, such as betamethasone, to accelerate differentiation of surfactant-secreting type II cells in the developing lungs. This acceleration of functional maturation of the fetal lungs decreases the incidence and severity of RDS in the newborn.

Premature Rupture of Membranes (PROM)

- PROM occurs when the amniotic sac ruptures before the onset of labor.
- PROM occurs in 10 to 15% of all pregnancies.
- The major risk of PROM is preterm labor and delivery. About 5% of patients with PROM will give birth preterm.
- Another common complication of PROM is chorioamnionitis, which has an increased incidence with earlier gestational age and positive cervical cultures for group B *streptococcus* (GBS) and *Neisseria gonorrhoeae*.
- PROM is diagnosed by a history of fluid leakage from the vagina and by examination with a sterile speculum.
- The nitrazine test measures fluid pH to distinguish amniotic fluid from urine and vaginal secretions. Nitrazine paper turns positive (dark blue) in response to alkaline amniotic fluid, cervical mucus, blood, and semen.
- "Ferning" is also used to distinguish amniotic fluid from other fluids. Ferning is the pattern of arborization that occurs when amniotic fluid is allowed to dry on a

slide. Ultrasound can also be used to evaluate the volume of amniotic fluid surrounding the fetus.

- During sterile speculum examination, cervical cultures for *Neisseria gonorrhoeae*, group B *streptococcus*, and *Chlamydia* are obtained. Amniotic fluid can also be tested for phosphatidylglycerol (PG), an indicator of fetal lung maturity.

- In order to decrease the risk of infection, intracervical digital examination should be avoided unless the patient is in active labor.

- If the evaluation suggests intrauterine infection, or the mother is febrile or septic, antibiotic therapy and delivery are indicated. Treat the infection with ampicillin, gentamicin, and metronidazole or clindamycin. Do not give tocolytics.

- If the fetus is significantly preterm and there is no evidence of infection, choose expectant management.

- If the fetus is at least 36 weeks, wait a few hours before inducing labor. If the fetus is at 35 weeks or less, wait 16 hours before inducing labor to promote lung maturation, then give the infant surfactant at birth.

- Betamethasone can also be given to promote fetal lung maturity. Prophylactic antibiotics should be given if the fetus is at 36 weeks or less.

Placenta Previa

- *CLASSIC PRESENTATION:* A pregnant woman in her third trimester who presents with the sudden onset of moderate vaginal bleeding. There is no pain or other symptom associated with the vaginal bleeding.

- Placenta previa refers to an abnormal location of the placenta over, or in close proximity to, the internal cervical os.

- Increasing maternal age, high parity, and previous C-sections are risk factors for placenta previa.

- Transabdominal ultrasound to diagnose placenta previa should be the first step in evaluating any pregnant woman with third trimester bleeding. A pelvic examination may precipitate massive hemorrhage in patients with placenta previa.

- Treatment includes hospitalization with hemodynamic stabilization or strict bedrest and pelvic rest until fetal lung maturity is attained. Magnesium sulfate is used to control uterine contractions.

- Cesarean delivery is almost always indicated.

- Placenta previa accreta is a further complication involving abnormal adherence of the placenta to the myometrium. At delivery, sustained and significant bleeding may occur and may require hysterectomy.

Abruptio Placentae

- *CLASSIC PRESENTATION:* A pregnant woman in the third trimester who presents with painful vaginal bleeding, lower abdominal and back discomfort, and painful uterine contractions. On examination she has a rigid, "board-like," tender uterus.

- Abruptio placentae, or placental abruption, refers to the premature separation of the normally implanted placenta from the uterine wall.

- Risk factors for placental abruption include hypertension, previous abruption, trauma, cocaine use, and smoking. Placental abruption may also be caused by the sudden decompression of the uterus in cases of rupture of membranes in patients with polyhydramnios or after delivery of the first of multiple fetuses.

- Diagnosis must be timely and is based on history, a tender uterus, and uterine contractions with some evidence of fetal distress. Ultrasound is of little benefit in diagnosing abruption, but it can exclude placenta previa as a cause for bleeding.

- The mother and the fetus may die of hemorrhage, and further contractions may worsen the abruption.

- Abruption is also the most common cause of consumptive coagulopathy in pregnancy; therefore, transfusions should be given to those patients requiring it with close follow-up of the coagulation status.

- Management includes hemodynamic stabilization and delivery. Delivery can be postponed while awaiting fetal lung maturity if there is limited abruption and no fetal or maternal distress. Any evidence of distress is an indication for immediate C-section.

Vasa Previa

- *CLASSIC PRESENTATION:* A pregnant woman in her third trimester who presents with a small amount of painless vaginal bleeding without other associated symptoms. Fetal tachycardia is noted during fetal monitoring. There is no evidence of placenta previa on ultrasound.

- Vasa previa is a rare condition in which the umbilical cord inserts into the membranes of the placenta rather than into the center of the placental tissue, and at least one vessel lies below the presenting fetal part near the internal os. If this vessel ruptures, fetal bleeding occurs and the fetus is at significant risk.

- A Betke-Kleihauer test may be done to distinguish fetal blood from maternal blood.

- Treatment requires immediate C-section to save the fetus.

Multiple Gestation

- The overall incidence of recognized twin gestation in the U.S. is approximately 1 in 90. Dizygotic (fraternal) twins occur when two separate ova are fertilized by two separate sperm, representing two siblings who happen to be born at the same time. Monozygotic (identical) twins are the result of the division of a fertilized ovum at various times after conception.

- Increased age and increased parity are risk factors for dizygotic twinning. A familial factor follows the maternal lineage.

- The likelihood of multiple gestation is significantly increased with the use of fertility agents and assisted reproduction.

- Only about 50% of twin pregnancies detected in the first trimester will result in the delivery of viable twins. Both spontaneous abortions and congenital anomalies occur more frequently in multiple pregnancies.
- As the number of fetuses increases, the expected duration of pregnancy decreases. Twins deliver at an average of 37 weeks.
- Multiple pregnancy is associated with increased perinatal morbidity. Significant causes of morbidity include preterm labor and delivery, intrauterine growth retardation, polyhydramnios, preeclampsia, congenital anomalies, and placental and umbilical cord accidents.

Uterine Rupture

- *CLASSIC PRESENTATION:* A pregnant woman in her third trimester who presents with the sudden onset of intense abdominal pain, with or without vaginal bleeding. There usually is a history of abdominal trauma.
- Risk factors include prior C-sections, trauma, and uterine distension.

Postterm Pregnancy

- A patient who has not delivered by the end of the week 42 is considered postterm. This occurs in 8 to 10% of pregnancies and recurs more often in patients with previous postterm pregnancies.
- Postterm newborns are at increased risk of dysmaturity, or postmaturity syndrome, in which affected infants are often growth retarded and have a loss of subcutaneous fat. Postterm newborns are often macrosomic (weighing >4000 g).
- These infants are at risk for hypoglycemia and hyperbilirubinemia. They have an increased risk of birth trauma secondary to their size.
- Postterm pregnancy is also associated with oligohydramnios, placental dysfunction, and meconium aspiration syndrome, which can lead to severe respiratory distress in the newborn.
- If pregnancy dates are demonstrably accurate, most postterm pregnancies will be induced by either 42 or 43 weeks.

SEXUALLY TRANSMITTED AND INFECTIOUS DISEASES DURING PREGNANCY

Bacterial Vaginosis

- Bacterial vaginosis should be treated with vaginal clindamycin or vaginal (NOT oral) metronidazole during pregnancy.

Chlamydia

- *Chlamydia* should be diagnosed early in pregnancy and treated with erythromycin, not doxycycline or tetracycline (contraindicated).

- More than one half of all infants born to women with cervical *Chlamydia trachomatis* are infected.
- Infants are at risk for conjunctivitis and pneumonia and their eyes should be treated prophylactically with erythromycin or silver nitrate.

Genital Herpes
- If lesions are present at the time of delivery, C-section is indicated to reduce the risk of fetal infection.

Gonorrhea
- Maternal infection with *Neisseria gonorrhoeae* causes neonatal ophthalmia.
- Bacteremia and arthritis result less commonly.
- Mothers should be treated with ceftriaxone during pregnancy.

Syphilis
- Maternal infection with *Treponema pallidum* causes congenital syphilis, which may result from any stage of maternal syphilis during pregnancy. There is an increased risk if the mother has early (primary or secondary) syphilis.
- Treat the mother with penicillin.

Trichomonas
- Metronidazole is contraindicated during the first trimester, but can be used cautiously thereafter.
- Vaginal metronidazole is recommended.

Group B *Streptococcus*
- Group B *Streptococcus* is commonly found in the vagina.
- Group B *Streptococcus* can cause neonatal sepsis and/or meningitis.
- Symptomatic babies are given ampicillin after birth.
- Mothers with prolonged rupture of membranes are also given ampicillin prophylaxis for possible group B *Streptococcus*.
- Vaginal cultures for group B *Streptococcus* are routinely taken during the third trimester, and affected mothers are treated with penicillin during labor.

Hepatitis B
- If the mother is positive for hepatitis B surface antigen, the baby should receive the hepatitis B vaccine and hyperimmune globulin at birth.

Human immunodeficiency Virus (HIV)
- Pregnant women infected with the HIV should receive AZT during the last two trimesters and during delivery.

- AZT reduces maternal-fetal transmission from 25% to less than 10%.
- The baby should receive AZT for the first 6 weeks of life.
- HIV testing should be encourage in all at-risk mothers during the first trimester of pregnancy.

LABOR AND DELIVERY

Normal Labor

- True labor is defined as the progressive effacement and dilation of the cervix, resulting from uterine contractions.
- False labor, or Braxton Hicks contractions, are uterine contractions without effacement and dilation of the cervix that occur normally during the third trimester.
- Patients should come to the hospital if contractions occur approximately every 5 minutes for at least 1 hour, if they feel a sudden or constant leakage of vaginal fluid, if there is any significant vaginal bleeding, or if there is decreased fetal movement.
- Labor is divided into four stages
  - **Stage 1**   From the onset of labor to full cervical dilation (10 cm). The latent phase is from cervical effacement and early dilation to 3 to 4 cm dilation. The active phase is from 3 to 4 cm dilation to full dilation. This phase is more rapid.
  - **Stage 2**   From complete cervical dilation through delivery of baby.
  - **Stage 3**   From the end of delivery of the baby through delivery of the placenta.
  - **Stage 4**   The immediate postpartum period of physiological adjustment and recovery of the mother, usually lasting about 2 hours.
- Fetal station is the relative level of the foremost presenting part of the fetus (usually the head) to the level of the ischial spines.
  1. If the presenting part is at the level of the spines, it is said to be at 0 station.
  2. If the presenting part is 3 cm below the ischial spines, it is said to be at +3 station.
  3. If the presenting part is 3 cm above the ischial spine, it is at -3 station.
- At 0 station, the greatest diameter of the fetal skull (biparietal diameter) has negotiated the pelvic inlet.
- The likelihood of serious postpartum complications is the greatest during the first hour or so after delivery.

Fetal Heart Monitoring During Labor

- Early heart rate decelerations are a vagal response to head compression and are normal during the second stage of labor. They do not indicate fetal distress.
- Late decelerations indicate uteroplacental insufficiency and fetal distress. The mother should be laid on her left side and given oxygen and subsequently, the baby should be delivered as soon as possible.
- Variable decelerations are a sign of umbilical cord compression. The mother should be laid on her left side and given oxygen by face mask. If the fetal heart rate continues to have variable decelerations, the baby should be delivered.

Abnormal Labor (Dystocia)

- Abnormally slow progress of labor is called a protraction disorder.
- Cessation of labor is called an arrest disorder.
- Cephalopelvic disproportion occurs when the fetal head is larger than the pelvis, preventing vaginal delivery. Cephalopelvic disproportion and shoulder dystocia (difficulty with delivery of the baby's shoulders) are often problems with large babies.
- The risks of prolonged labor include:
  1. Maternal: infection, exhaustion, lacerations, and uterine atony with possible hemorrhage.
  2. Fetal: asphyxia, trauma, infection, cerebral damage secondary to prolonged pressure on the head, and meconium aspiration syndrome.
- The management of dystocia can include induction of labor, augmentation of labor by stimulation of the uterine cervix, artificial rupture of membranes, and delivery using forceps, vacuum, or C-section.
- In the face of fetal or maternal distress, C-section should always be used unless the mother is in the second stage of labor with the vertex low in the pelvis, in which case forceps or vacuum delivery can be attempted.

Breech Presentation

- Breech presentation occurs in 2 to 4% of term pregnancies, and a higher percentage of preterm deliveries.
- Risk factors for breech presentation include prematurity, multiple gestation, polyhydramnios, hydrocephaly, anencephaly, uterine anomalies and uterine tumors.
- The diagnosis of breech presentation is made by Leopold's maneuvers and ultrasound.
- The different types of breech presentation are as follows:
  1. frank breech - buttocks first, legs straight up by head
  2. complete breech - buttocks and feet first
  3. incomplete breech - buttocks and one foot first, or foot first

- Breech deliveries have an increased morbidity and mortality for both the mother and baby.
- Management can include external cephalic version and/or C-section.
- Frank breech can sometimes be delivered vaginally.

Gestational Trophoblastic Neoplasia/ Molar Pregnancy

- *CLASSIC PRESENTATION:* A woman early in the second trimester of pregnancy who presents with painless vaginal bleeding with a positive pregnancy test and often a uterine size/date discrepancy. She may also have severe nausea and vomiting, visual disturbances, preeclampsia, and proteinuria. Ultrasound examination reveals a characteristic "snowstorm" appearance of molar pregnancy.
- Gestational trophoblastic neoplasia is a rare variation of pregnancy that in most instances is a benign disease called molar pregnancy (hydatidiform mole). These neoplasms are derived from abnormal placental (trophoblastic) proliferation. Fewer than 10% of patients with molar pregnancy will develop persistent or malignant disease.
- A complete mole contains no fetus and accounts for approximately 90% of all molar pregnancies.
- An incomplete mole contains a fetus plus molar degeneration.
- Upon diagnosis, the level of β-hCG is extremely high in molar pregnancy and can help both to classify risk category and to serve as a sensitive tumor marker for further follow-up.
- Treatment consists of prompt surgical removal of the intrauterine contents. Patients must then be followed closely for at least 1 year with periodic pelvic examination and quantitative hCG levels.
- Failure of quantitative hCG levels to regress suggests recurrent benign gestational trophoblastic neoplasia and/or malignant transformation to choriocarcinoma, occurring in less than 10% of patients. Treatment for this is usually chemotherapy.
- The recurrence rate of molar pregnancy is 2%.

POSTPARTUM COMPLICATIONS

Postpartum Hemorrhage

- Postpartum hemorrhage is defined as greater than 500 mL of blood loss during and after delivery.
- This occurs in about 1% of patients.
- Postpartum hemorrhage is more likely to occur in cases of rapid labor, prolonged labor, uterine enlargement (large baby, polyhydramnios, uterine leiomyoma), or with the use of drugs that inhibit uterine contraction.
- Uterine atony is by far the most common cause of postpartum hemorrhage. Genital tract trauma (obstetrical lacerations) are the next most common cause.

- Management includes uterine massage and oxytocin infusion in intravenous fluids to promote uterine contraction.
- If bleeding continues, the uterus may be explored to look for retained products of conception and then packed with gauze. Methergine and prostaglandin preparations may be used to promote vasoconstriction and uterine contraction.
- If bleeding continues, surgical management may include arterial ligation or embolization and/or hysterectomy.

Puerperal Febrile Morbidity

- Puerperal febrile morbidity is defined as a temperature of greater than 38° C (100.4° F) occurring on any 2 of the first 10 days postpartum, exclusive of the first 24 hours. However, even fevers during the first 24-hour postpartum are generally thought to represent infection.
- The most common source of postpartum infection is metritis (endometrial inflammation), which is usually associated with the development of fever on the first or second day postpartum. There is often uterine and/or adnexal tenderness on postpartum examination.
- The infection is usually polymicrobial and is treated on clinical suspicion, usually without cultures.
- Ampicillin and gentamicin or a cephalosporin such as cefotetan may be used. Antibiotics are continued until the patient is asymptomatic, has normal bowel function, and has been afebrile for at least 24 hours.
- Other common sources of postpartum fevers are atelectasis, UTI, wound infections, and mastitis.
- An uncommon infection and sequela of pelvic infection is septic pelvic thrombophlebitis. This occurs when venous stasis in the pelvic veins, along with the presence of bacteria, lead to septic thrombosis in these vessels and to microembolization of the lungs or other organs.
- The symptoms of septic pelvic thrombophlebitis are residual fever and tachycardia following several days of antibiotics for metritis.
- The treatment of septic pelvic thrombophlebitis is empiric heparin for 7 to 30 days.
- Resolution of the fever and tachycardia within the next few days supports the diagnosis.

NOTES

Chapter 3

GYNECOLOGY

Susan L. Taylor, M.D.

CONTRACEPTION

Oral Contraceptives

- Oral contraceptives (OCs) are a very effective method of contraception with compliant patients. Failure rates are less than 1%.
- Oral contraceptive users have an increased risk of deep-vein thrombosis (DVT), myocardial infarction, and hemorrhagic stroke but a decreased risk of endometrial and ovarian cancer.
- Absolute contraindications for OCs include liver tumors, breast cancer, pregnancy, heart disease, thromboembolic disease, cerebrovascular disease, and estrogen-dependent tumors.
- Oral contraceptives should not be used in over 35-year-old smokers due to increased risk of cardiovascular disease.

Long-acting Hormonal Methods

- Injectable (Depo-Provera) and implantable (Norplant), long-acting hormonal methods of contraception are highly effective without concern for daily compliance.
- Both of these progestin methods act to suppress ovulation, thicken cervical mucus, and alter the rate of ovum transport to prevent pregnancy.

Barrier Methods

- Barrier contraceptives, such as condoms, diaphragms, and cervical caps, depend on proper use before or at the time of intercourse and are subject to a higher failure rate than oral contraceptives.
- Condoms are the only method of contraception that provide protection against sexually transmitted diseases, specifically HIV. However, they still do not provide complete protection.

Intrauterine Devices

- Intrauterine contraceptive devices (IUDs) are inserted into the endometrial cavity and can remain in place for up to several years. They act to prevent implantation of the conceptus.
- IUDs are effective but have a high rate of complications including uterine perforation, spontaneous expulsion, ectopic pregnancies, pelvic infections, menorrhagia, and menstrual pain.
- IUDs should be used in women who are at low risk for sexually transmitted diseases (STDs) and do not desire to have any more children.

Tubal Ligation

- Tubal ligation is an effective method of sterilization, but it is not 100% effective. The pregnancy rate is less than 1%.

- Patients have an increased proportion of ectopic pregnancies if they become pregnant.

Vasectomy
- Vasectomy is an effective method of sterilization, with a pregnancy rate of about 1%. Vasectomy is more easily reversed than most female sterilization procedures.
- Semen analysis should confirm the absence of sperm prior to sexual intercourse.

BREAST DISORDERS

Benign Breast Disorders
- Fibrocystic changes present as cyclic, bilateral mastalgia, and engorgement.
- Fibroadenoma presents as a firm, painless, freely movable breast lump. The lump is slow growing and does not change with the menstrual cycle. This is very common in young women.
- Intraductal papilloma presents with spontaneous bloody, serous, or cloudy nipple discharge usually without a palpable mass. Papillomas arise in the ducts of the breast and are the most common cause of bloody nipple discharge.
- Mammary duct ectasia usually presents in the fifth decade of life with thick gray to black nipple discharge, as well as nipple pain and tenderness. It is caused by chronic intraductal and periductal inflammation leading to obstruction and dilation of the ducts by secretions.

Breast Cancer
- CLASSIC PRESENTATION: A woman over the age of 40 who presents with a painless breast mass. There may be nipple discharge and skin changes such as *peau d'orange* (orange peel skin), which are late symptoms associated with a poor prognosis.
- The risk factors of breast cancer include age, a first-degree relative with breast or ovarian cancer, early menarche, late menopause, and nulliparity. Only about 20% of 30- to 54-year-old patients with breast cancer are identified by risk factors.
- Eighty percent of breast cancers are of the nonspecific infiltrating intraductal type.
- The diagnosis is made by imaging with mammography and ultrasound. Use fine-needle aspiration (FNA) or open biopsy for tissue diagnosis.
- Breast cancer therapy is based on the stage of disease, the number of axillary lymph nodes affected, and the presence of hormone receptors.
- Treatment is usually surgical with adjunctive treatment (including radiation, chemotherapy, hormonal therapy, or a combination of these).
- Tamoxifen citrate is an estrogen receptor antagonist that is used as adjunctive therapy for estrogen receptor positive breast cancers.

- Mammography guidelines: Women should have a baseline mammogram before age 40, mammograms every 1 to 2 years between age 40 and 50, and a yearly mammogram after age 50. Mammograms are obtained more frequently for some women with a positive history or family history of breast cancer, or for diagnostic purposes when a lump is felt.

COMMON GYNECOLOGICAL PROBLEMS

Dysmenorrhea

- *CLASSIC PRESENTATION:* A woman who presents with the complaint of painful menstruation. The patient may note crampy lower abdominal pain that may be accompanied by nausea, vomiting, diarrhea, fatigue, backaches, and headaches.
- Primary dysmenorrhea is caused by an excess of prostaglandins leading to painful uterine muscle activity.
- Primary dysmenorrhea usually presents as recurrent, spasmodic lower abdominal pain on the first 1 to 3 days of menstruation.
- Secondary dysmenorrhea is caused by some other clinically identifiable cause.
- The treatment of dysmenorrhea includes NSAIDS, exercise, heat, and sometimes oral contraceptives to prevent ovulation.

Amenorrhea

- If a woman has never menstruated, she has primary amenorrhea. If a woman has previously menstruated but has not menstruated within 6 months, she has secondary amenorrhea. If she has not menstruated for more than 1 but less than 6 months, she has oligomenorrhea.
- Amenorrhea indicates a failure to ovulate.
- Causes of amenorrhea include pregnancy (most common), hypothalamic-pituitary dysfunction, ovarian failure, obstruction of the genital outflow tract, weight loss, or drug abuse.
- Women with amenorrhea and no genital tract anomalies are in a state of estrogen deficiency.
- In considering a diagnosis for the cause of amenorrhea, first do a pregnancy test. Then consider tests such as FSH and prolactin levels. A hysterosalpingogram may be performed to look for genital tract obstruction.
- If hyperprolactinemia secondary to a pituitary adenoma is the cause of the amenorrhea, the treatment is bromocriptine, a dopamine agonist.
- Treat premature ovarian failure (i.e., early menopause) with exogenous estrogen replacement.

Endometriosis

- *CLASSIC PRESENTATION:* A 20- to 30-year-old woman with dysmenorrhea, pelvic pain, abnormal bleeding, deep thrust dyspareunia, and/or infertility. She has tried oral contraceptives to help her pain without response. Pelvic examination reveals mild adnexal tenderness. There is uterosacral nodularity on rectovaginal examination.

- Endometriosis is defined as the presence of endometrial tissue in extrauterine locations, most commonly the ovaries. The uterosacral ligaments, pelvic peritoneum, and rectovaginal septum are other common sites. This is a progressive disease.

- A diagnosis is made by laparoscopy or laparotomy.

- Treatment: Expectant management if the disease is limited and fertility is important. Limited disease can also be treated by oral contraceptives, danazol (suppresses LH and FSH), or GnRH agonists.

- Surgery is the only treatment for extensive disease or disease that is unresponsive to medical therapies.

Dysfunctional Uterine Bleeding

- Irregular uterine bleeding also indicates a failure to ovulate. Women with dysfunctional uterine bleeding are in a state of chronic estrogen stimulation.

- The most common causes are polycystic ovarian disease, exogenous obesity, and adrenal hyperplasia.

- Dysfunctional uterine bleeding can also occur with a luteal phase defect, a condition in which the patient has a shortened menstrual cycle because the corpus luteum is unable to support the endometrium for the usual 13 to 14 days and is unable to support a pregnancy.

- In making a diagnosis, anatomical causes such as uterine leiomyomata, inflammation or infection of the cervix or vagina, cervical or endometrial carcinoma, cervical erosions or polyps, and vaginal lesions must be excluded. Polycystic ovarian disease is a diagnosis of exclusion.

- Treatment consists of oral contraceptives or intermittent progesterone.

Candida Vaginitis

- *CLASSIC PRESENTATION:* A woman with a complaint of vulvar or vaginal itching, burning, external dysuria, and/or dyspareunia, accompanied by a thick, adherent, "cottage cheese-like", odorless vaginal discharge.

- Candidiasis is usually caused by *C. albicans* (yeast) and more likely to occur in women who are pregnant, diabetic, obese, immunocompromised, taking oral contraceptives or corticosteroids, or who have recently had broad-spectrum antibiotics.

- Treatment is primarily with topical application of a synthetic imidazole, or a single dose of the oral agent fluconazole.

- Partners are not treated because candidal infections are not usually sexually transmitted.

Atrophic Vaginitis

- *CLASSIC PRESENTATION:* A postmenopausal woman with complaints of vaginal dryness during sexual intercourse, vaginal itching and burning, and diminished sexual enjoyment.
- Treatment with estrogen replacement therapy restores the integrity of the vaginal epithelium, relieving symptoms of vaginal dryness, itching, and dyspareunia.

Other Types of Vaginitis

- When a woman presents with vaginitis, also consider bacterial vaginitis and *Trichomonas vaginalis* infection (see Sexually Transmitted Diseases section).

SEXUALLY TRANSMITTED DISEASES

Bacterial Vaginosis

- *CLASSIC PRESENTATION:* A woman with a complaint of a thin gray-white vaginal discharge that has a "musty" or "fishy" odor.
- Mixing of vaginal discharge with KOH ("whiff test") will liberate amines and cause a distinct fishy odor.
- Saline wet mount reveals a slight increase in WBCs, characteristic "clue cells" (epithelial cells with numerous bacilli on their surface, making them appear to have indistinct borders) and often clumps of bacteria.
- Treat with metronidazole or clindamycin. Treat sexual partners.

Trichomoniasis

- *CLASSIC PRESENTATION:* A woman with a complaint of a "frothy," thin, yellow-green to gray vaginal discharge with a rancid odor, often accompanied by vulvar itching or burning, dysuria, and/or dyspareunia.
- Wet mount reveals large numbers of WBCs and the *Trichomonas* organism, a flagellate protozoan that is slightly larger than a WBC.
- Treatment is with metronidazole. Treat sexual partners.

Herpes Genitalis

- *CLASSIC PRESENTATION:* A patient with a prodromal phase of paresthesias (e.g., burning) a few days after sexual intercourse, followed by the development of painful, clear, vesicular and ulcerated lesions around the genital area within the next 3 to 7 days.
- Eighty-five percent of lesions are caused by HSV-2. Fifteen percent of lesions are caused by HSV-1, which usually causes the "cold sore" lesions in the mouth.
- Herpes simplex virus is highly contagious and produces a recurrent infection.
- Viral cultures can confirm the diagnosis, as can a Wright stain.

- Treatment is with acyclovir, which is effective in decreasing both the frequency and severity of flare-ups.

Gonorrhea
- *Neisseria gonorrhoeae* is a Gram-negative, intracellular coccus causing cervicitis, salpingitis, pelvic inflammatory disease, perihepatitis (Fitz-Hugh and Curtis syndrome), polyarthritis, and pharyngitis.
- Diagnosis is made by culture on Thayer-Martin agar.
- Treatment is ceftriaxone plus doxycycline for presumed chlamydial coinfection.

Chlamydia
- *Chlamydia trachomatis* is an obligate intracellular parasite causing cervicitis, acute urethritis, salpingitis, pelvic inflammatory disease, lymphogranuloma venereum, and perihepatitis (Fitz-Hugh and Curtis syndrome).
- A diagnosis of chlamydial infection is made by cervical culture.
- Treat suspected or confirmed patients with infections and their partners with doxycycline.

Pelvic Inflammatory Disease (PID)
- PID is an infection of the upper female genital tract, usually caused by direct spread from initial infection of the cervix.
- *Chlamydia trachomatis* and *Neisseria gonorrhoeae* are the most common organisms causing PID.
- Anaerobes thrive in the female reproductive tract and often cause a polymicrobial infection.
- PID should be treated aggressively, often with hospitalization and IV antibiotic therapy if indicated.

Human Papilloma Virus (HPV)
- HPV is a DNA virus that causes condyloma acuminata or venereal warts.
- At least 3 subtypes of HPV (16, 18, and 31) have been associated with the development of cervical neoplasia.
- Treat HPV with podophyllin, cryosurgery, electrodesiccation, surgical excision, or laser vaporization.

Syphilis
- *CLASSIC PRESENTATION:* A sexually active patient with a painless chancre on the genitalia.
- Syphilis is caused by the spirochete *Treponema pallidum*.
- Primary syphilis is the development of a painless ulcer, called a chancre, about 10 to 60 days after infection.

- Four to 8 weeks after the chancre appears, manifestations of secondary syphilis develop, including low-grade fevers, headache, malaise, sore throat, generalized lymphadenopathy, and a diffuse, symmetric maculopapular rash that characteristically covers the palms and soles.
- Condyloma lata may form on the vulva, and are distinguished from venereal warts by their flat-top appearance.
- The disease then enters a latent phase, and can then emerge as tertiary syphilis, which can cause crippling damage to the central nervous system, heart, or great vessels.
- Diagnosis is by serologic testing for VDRL or RPR, which can be confirmed by the more specific tests FTA-ABS and MHA-TP.
- The treatment of choice for syphilis is penicillin G.

Human Immunodeficiency Virus (HIV) / Acquired Immunodeficiency Syndrome (AIDS)

- Please refer to the Internal Medicine chapter.

COMMON GYNECOLOGIC ISSUES

Infertility
- Infertility is defined as failure to conceive after 1 year of unprotected sex.
- Forty percent of infertility is due to male dysfunction. Sperm quality is assessed by volume and evaluation of fresh semen.
- The most common cause of female infertility is endometriosis. Other common causes are tubal occlusion secondary to PID or adhesions, anovulation, and anatomical disorders of the female genital tract.
- Ovulatory status may be evaluated by recording basal body temperatures.
- The genital tract may be evaluated anatomically with hysterosalpingography.
- Endometriosis is diagnosed by laparoscopy or laparotomy.
- Treatment: Anovulation can be treated with clomiphene citrate (an antiestrogen) or FSH. In some cases of infertility, artificial insemination or assisted reproductive techniques are used.

Menopause
- Menopause is defined as the cessation of menses due to ovarian failure. The mean age of menopause is 50 years. Menopause is called premature if it occurs before age 42.
- The climacteric is the period of waning ovarian function occurring before menopause.

- Perimenopausal women have symptoms of menstrual irregularity, sleep disturbances, emotional changes, and hot flashes. After menopause, women experience atrophic vaginitis, osteoporosis, and increased atherosclerosis.
- Menopause occurs as the ovaries become less responsive to FSH and LH.
- Treatment consists of estrogen replacement therapy to diminish the signs and symptoms of ovarian failure and maintain bone mass and plasma lipids at normal levels. If the woman has a uterus, administer the estrogen with a progestin to prevent the effects of unopposed estrogen on the uterus (endometrial hyperplasia and adenocarcinoma).

Hirsutism and Virilization

- *CLASSIC PRESENTATION:* A woman with hirsutism has excess body hair, usually manifested initially as midline dark, coarse hair on the lower abdomen, around the nipples, and around the chin and upper lip. Acne is also common. Virilization is masculinization that manifests by enlargement of the clitoris, temporal balding, deepening of the voice, and breast involution.
- Hirsutism and virilization are signs of androgen excess.
- The most common cause of hirsutism is polycystic ovarian disease. The second most common cause is adrenal hyperplasia.
- Other causes of hirsutism and virilization include hyperthecosis, androgen-secreting tumors (Sertoli-Leydig cell tumors), congenital adrenal hyperplasia (21-hydroxylase deficiency), adrenal neoplasms, and iatrogenic androgen excess.
- Congenital adrenal hyperplasia, in its most severe form, presents as a virilized newborn female infant.

COMMON OVARIAN PROBLEMS

Functional Ovarian Cysts

- *CLASSIC PRESENTATION:* A premenopausal woman with mild to severe unilateral lower abdominal pain and alteration of the menstrual interval. Pelvic examination findings may include unilateral adnexal tenderness with a palpable, mobile, cystic adnexal mass.
- A follicular cyst develops when an ovarian follicle fails to rupture during follicular maturation and ovulation does not occur. This causes a lengthening of the follicular phase with secondary amenorrhea. Follicular cysts usually resolve spontaneously, but on occasion may rupture and cause acute pelvic pain.
- Diagnosis: A pregnancy test must be performed first to rule out ectopic pregnancy. Pelvic ultrasound is usually not required if the cyst is less than 5 cm in diameter and the patient can be reassured and followed with a repeat pelvic examination in 6 to 8 weeks.

- In patients with larger cysts, pelvic ultrasound may be warranted, and this may reveal a unilocular simple cyst without blood or soft tissue elements.
- Treatment: Most follicular cysts spontaneously resolve in 6 to 8 weeks. Alternatively, oral contraceptives may be given to suppress gonadotropin stimulation of the cyst.
- If the cyst persists, the presence of another type of cyst or neoplasm should be suspected. In persistent cysts, further radiological studies and/or surgery may be indicated.
- Another common type of functional ovarian cyst is a corpus luteum cyst, which is related to the postovulatory phase of the menstrual cycle.
- Persistent corpus luteum cysts are often associated with dull lower quadrant pain, missed menses with a negative pregnancy test, and adnexal enlargement.
- Treatment is usually not necessary, but patients with recurrent persistent corpus luteum cysts may benefit from cyclic OCs.

Polycystic Ovarian Disease (PCOD)

- *CLASSIC PRESENTATION:* An overweight young woman with oligomenorrhea or amenorrhea, anovulation, acne, hirsutism, and/or infertility.
- PCOD is caused by obesity, genetic predisposition, and other causes of LH excess.
- The connection of PCOD to obesity occurs through the following mechanism:
    1. Luteinizing hormone (LH) normally stimulates the theca lutein cells in the ovaries to increase androstenedione and testosterone production.
    2. Androstenedione is converted to estrone (a weak estrogen) in fat cells.
    3. Estrone has a stimulating effect on the pituitary secretion of LH.
    4. With obesity, there are more fat cells to convert androstenedione to estrone.
    5. The increased estrone then stimulates increased LH secretion, which leads to further androstenedione and testosterone production.
    6. The increased testosterone levels cause the acne and hirsutism associated with polycystic ovarian disease.
- This is a functional disorder of androgen excess that is treated with weight reduction and oral contraceptives.

URINARY INCONTINENCE

General

- Almost 50% of all women have had the involuntary loss of a few drops of urine at some point in their life, and 10 to 15% of women suffer significant, recurrent loss.
- Mostly as a result of aging, pelvic relaxation can cause problems of urinary incontinence, pelvic pressure and pain, dyspareunia, and bowel dysfunction.
- Urinary incontinence is a common complaint of patients with a cystocele (descent or prolapse of the bladder) or urethrocele (descent or prolapse of the urethra).

- Diagnosis: The degree of pelvic relaxation is best evaluated by vaginal examination while the patient strains. The presence of a cystocele, rectocele, or enterocele may be observed, as well as degree of uterine prolapse.
- A urethrocele may be evaluated using the cotton swab test, in which a cotton swab is placed in the urethra and the angle of upward motion caused by the patient straining is measured. Upward rotation of greater than 30 degrees from the starting point is associated with urinary stress incontinence.
- Urodynamics testing may also be used to evaluate bladder structure and function.

Stress Incontinence

- *CLASSIC PRESENTATION:* A patient with the complaint of small spurts of urine being lost with stress events such as coughing, laughing, sneezing, and physical activity.
- Stress incontinence often has a structural cause such as a cystocele or urethrocele.
- The treatment includes Kegel's exercises to strengthen the pelvic musculature, surgical measures, and/or pessaries for mechanical vaginal support.

Urge Incontinence

- *CLASSIC PRESENTATION:* A patient with the complaint of the complete emptying of the bladder without any associated event or change in position. It may also be associated with urgency and nocturia.
- The cause is loss of bladder inhibition.
- Treatment includes bladder training, biofeedback, and often anticholinergics, β-agonists, and/or antidepressants.

Overflow Incontinence

- *CLASSIC PRESENTATION:* A patient with the complaint of continuous dribbling of small amounts of urine, associated with a feeling of bladder fullness or pressure.
- Overflow incontinence is caused by loss of neurologic control of the bladder or obstruction of the urinary tract.
- Diagnose and treat any causes of urinary tract obstruction.
- Treatment of neurologic causes is supportive.

GYNECOLOGIC NEOPLASMS

Vulvar Cancer

- *CLASSIC PRESENTATION:* A postmenopausal female with vulvar pruritus, burning, nonspecific irritation, and/or the feeling of a vulvar mass. Physical examination reveals a red or white exophytic or ulcerative lesion of the labia majora.
- Vulvar carcinoma represents about 4% of gynecological cancers. Ninety percent of vulvar cancers are of the squamous cell type.
- Diagnosis of vulvar cancer is made by biopsy. Any suspicious vulvar lesion, especially in an older woman, should be biopsied.
- Treatment is surgical removal with wide excision. The prognosis is good.

Vaginal Cancer

- *CLASSIC PRESENTATION:* A postmenopausal, asymptomatic woman who is found to have a red, ulcerated, or white hyperplastic lesion of the vagina.
- Vaginal carcinoma represents only 1 to 2% of gynecological cancers. Ninety five percent of vaginal carcinomas are of the squamous cell type. The rest are adenocarcinomas (such as clear cell adenocarcinoma, which is usually related to diethylstilbestrol (DES) exposure *in utero*) and vaginal melanoma.
- The diagnosis of vaginal cancer is usually by biopsy, although occasionally vaginal carcinoma is detected on Papanicolaou (Pap) smears of the vaginal mucosa.
- Radiation therapy is the mainstay of treatment for vaginal squamous cell carcinoma.
- Sarcoma botryoides (also known as embryonal rhabdomyosarcoma) presents as a mass of grape-like polyps protruding from the introitus of very young girls and infants.

Cervical Cancer

- *CLASSIC PRESENTATION:* A woman who presents with postcoital bleeding and/or abnormal uterine bleeding.
- This is the second most common malignancy in women. The death rate from cervical cancer has decreased in recent years due to early detection by Pap smears and subsequent treatment.
- Risk factors for cervical cancer include early sexual intercourse, multiple sexual partners, cigarette smoking, human papilloma virus infection, and immunosuppression.
- The Pap smear is used to diagnose squamous cell carcinoma of the cervix and its precursor lesions (cervical dysplasia).
- Abnormal Pap smears are followed by colposcopy with biopsy of suspicious areas and endocervical curettage.
- Treatment is radical surgery and/or pelvic irradiation. The precursor lesions of cervical dysplasia are treated by cervical conization, laser, loop excision, or electrical cauterization.

Uterine Leiomyomas (Fibroids)

- *CLASSIC PRESENTATION:* A pre- or postmenopausal woman with lower abdominal pain, abnormal vaginal bleeding, and/or symptoms related to pressure of the uterus against the bowel, bladder, or pelvic floor. Upon physical examination the patient has a "lumpy bumpy uterus."
- Vaginal bleeding is the most common presenting symptom.
- Up to 30% of American women have these benign tumors, and the majority of these women have few or no significant symptoms.
- A fibroid is a localized proliferation of smooth muscle cells surrounded by a pseudocapsule of muscle fibers. These tumors are hormonally responsive, and their growth is related to estrogen production.
- Menopause usually brings about cessation of growth and often even atrophy. However, the benign tumors may continue to grow with estrogen replacement therapy.
- In 0.1% to 1% of cases, malignancy (leiomyosarcoma) may occur. This should be suspected in postmenopausal women, especially if the tumor continues to increase in size without estrogen stimulation.
- The diagnosis is usually made by physical examination and ultrasound.
- Treatment is most often expectant management if there are few or no symptoms and the patient can be followed by serial physical and ultrasonographic examinations. If required, surgery can be myomectomy or hysterectomy.
- Fibroids are the most common indication for hysterectomy in the U.S.
- Treatment of leiomyosarcoma is usually total hysterectomy with bilateral salpingo-oophorectomy.

Endometrial Cancer

- *CLASSIC PRESENTATION:* A postmenopausal woman with abnormal uterine bleeding.
- Endometrial cancer is the most common female genital tract malignancy.
- The etiology of endometrial hyperplasia and endometrial cancer is overgrowth of the endometrium in response to an estrogen-dominant hormonal environment.
- Risk factors for endometrial carcinoma include any features contributing to an increased estrogen environment, such as obesity, patients using exogenous estrogen alone, late menopause, history of chronic anovulation, nulliparity, and diabetes mellitus.
- Diagnosis by endometrial biopsy is highly accurate and should be used liberally in women over age 35 presenting with abnormal uterine bleeding. Occasionally, atypical endometrial cells are found on the Pap smear, but this is not reliable in diagnosing endometrial cancer.
- Treatment for endometrial carcinoma is total abdominal hysterectomy with bilateral salpingo-oophorectomy, often with adjunctive radiation therapy.

- Treatment of simple hyperplasia, cystic hyperplasia, and adenomatous hyperplasia is usually medical with a short course of progestin each month. Treatment of atypical adenomatous hyperplasia, thought to be a true neoplastic process, is hysterectomy.

Ovarian Cancer

- *CLASSIC PRESENTATION:* A woman over the age of 40 who presents with a palpable adnexal mass and no other symptoms. Occasionally, a woman will present with increasing abdominal girth and a palpable abdominopelvic mass.
- Ovarian carcinoma is the third most common gynecologic malignancy but has the highest mortality rate of all the gynecologic malignancies, primarily because early detection before widespread dissemination is difficult.
- Ovarian neoplasms are usually only symptomatic after extensive metastasis, and there is no effective screening test for ovarian carcinoma.
- Risk factors for ovarian carcinoma include advancing age, low parity, decreased fertility, delayed childbearing, and positive family history.
- Long-term suppression of ovulation, such as oral contraceptive use, may be protective against the development of ovarian cancer.

Benign Ovarian Neoplasms

- In women of reproductive age, 90% of ovarian neoplasms are benign, whereas in postmenopausal women, the risk of malignancy is greater than 25%. Benign ovarian neoplasms are more common than malignant ovarian tumors in all age groups.
- Benign neoplasms have an increased chance of malignant transformation with increasing age and are treated surgically because of their risk for malignant transformation.
- The most common tumor found in women of all ages is the benign cystic teratoma, also called a dermoid cyst or dermoid. Dermoids are germ cell tumors and may contain differentiated tissue from all three embryonic germ layers. The most common elements found are skin appendages with associated hair follicles and sebum, as well as nervous tissue, cartilage, bone and teeth. An unusual variant, struma ovarii, contains functioning thyroid tissue.

Malignant Ovarian Neoplasms

- About 90% of malignant ovarian tumors are of the epithelial cell type, with the remainder being germ cell tumors and stromal cell tumors.
- Of the epithelial cell malignancies, the serous cystadenocarcinoma is the most common. About 30% of these are bilateral at the time of clinical presentation. Other epithelial cell malignancies are the mucinous cystadenocarcinoma, endometrioid tumors, clear cell carcinomas, and Brenner's tumors.
- Germ cell tumors constitute less than 5% of ovarian malignancies, but are the most common ovarian cancers in women under the age of 20. The most common germ cell malignancies are the dysgerminoma and immature teratoma. Rare germ cell tumors

include endodermal sinus tumors, which produce α-fetoprotein, and embryonal cell carcinoma, which produce both α-fetoprotein and β-hCG.

● Stromal cell malignant tumors are functional tumors because they produce hormones. The granulosa cell tumor may produce large amounts of estrogen. The Sertoli-Leydig cell tumor is a rare testosterone-secreting tumor that may present with hirsutism or virilization.

● A Krukenberg's tumor is an ovarian tumor that is metastatic from another site, most commonly from the GI tract (stomach especially) and breast.

● The diagnosis of all ovarian malignancies is histologic. Staging is surgical.

● The treatment of ovarian malignancies is usually by surgical removal with wide excision followed by chemotherapy and/or radiation depending on the stage and tumor type.

NOTES

Chapter 4

INTERNAL MEDICINE

Aamer H. Jamali, M.D.

PREVENTIVE MEDICINE

Causes of Death
- The leading causes of death in the U.S. (in order of prevalence) are heart disease, cancer, and stroke.
- Accidental death is the leading cause of death of the 1 to 25 age group.
- The leading cause of death for 25- to 44-year-olds was AIDS, but that has recently changed to accidental death.

Smoking Cessation
- The immediate benefits of smoking cessation include healing of peptic ulcers, decrease in cough, and decrease in phlegm production.
- Smoking cessation also will decrease the risk of thromboembolic phenomena (MI, stroke).
- There is no reversal of COPD with smoking cessation.
- Smoking cessation will decrease the risk of lung cancer up to 99%. There are also decreases in oral, esophageal, pancreatic, and bladder cancer with smoking cessation.

Cancer (CA) Prevention
- The most common cancers in men (in order of prevalence) are prostate, lung, and colon. In women, they are breast, colon, and lung.
- The most lethal cancers in men are lung, prostate, and colon. The most lethal cancers in women are lung, breast, and colon.
- Cervical CA can be treated with better success with early detection with Papanicolaou smears every year after age 18 or first coitus.
- Breast CA can be treated with better success with early detection with clinical breast examinations every year after age 18, and mammograms every 1 to 2 years after age 40 (controversial age 30 to 40).
- Colon CA can be treated with better success by testing for occult blood every year, and flexible sigmoidoscopy every 5 years after age 50.
- Prostate CA can be treated with better success with digital rectal examination yearly after age 50, consider PSA (controversial).
- Testicular CA is most common in young men. Regular testicular self-examination, ages 19 to 45 can lead to earlier detection.

Cardiovascular Disease Reduction
- Try lifestyle changes first, before medications, unless lipid elevations are severe. If smoking cessation is a choice, it is usually the correct first step. Try exercise, weight loss, and to a lesser extent, dietary restriction of fat and salt.
- Antihyperlipidemic drug therapy is a last resort.

VITAMIN DEFICIENCIES

Folate vs. Vitamin B$_{12}$ Deficiency

- For the purposes of Boards, note that most megaloblastic (macrocytic) anemia is due to one of these two deficiencies.
- Look for a time frame of the symptoms, since vitamin B$_{12}$ deficiency will take a matter of 4 to 5 years to develop.
- Look for the diet patterns described, since folate deficiency will be found in alcoholics, and vitamin B$_{12}$ deficiency will be found in strict vegetarians.
- Look for associated symptoms; vitamin B$_{12}$ deficiency is associated with polyneuropathy and atrophic glossitis, whereas folate deficiency does not have any associated neurological signs or symptoms.

Niacin Deficiency (Pellagra)

- *CLASSIC PRESENTATION:* A patient who presents with skin changes (photosensitivity), altered mental status, and diarrhea, often found in a person from the southern United States or Latin America.
- Remember the **three *D*'s**:
    *D*ermatitis
    *D*ementia
    *D*iarrhea.

Vitamin B$_6$ (Pyridoxine) Deficiency

- *CLASSIC PRESENTATION:* A patient who has been taking isoniazid (INH) for 6 months complains of sensory paresthesias in a stocking-glove distribution.
- Think of vitamin B$_6$ (pyridoxine) deficiency in a patient on INH, cyclosporine, or penicillamine therapy with a peripheral paresthesia/polyneuropathy.

Vitamin C Deficiency (Scurvy)

- *CLASSIC PRESENTATION:* A young infant receiving unsupplemented formula, or a middle-aged to elderly patient (usually male) presents originally with perifollicular papules and hemorrhages, which coalesce into purpura, which then advance to more severe hemorrhagic complications (ecchymoses, gum bleeding, and/or hemarthrosis).

Thiamine (Vitamin B$_1$) Deficiency

- Thiamine deficiency is found in alcoholics and those on hemodialysis and can result in beriberi (high output heart failure plus or minus peripheral neuropathy), Wernicke's syndrome which presents with cerebellar signs such as ataxia, and Korsakoff's syndrome which is associated with memory disturbances.

Total Parenteral Nutrition (TPN)-Related Deficiencies

- *CLASSIC PRESENTATION:* A patient on TPN who begins to experience alopecia, dermatitis, and diarrhea may have zinc deficiency. Zinc deficiency is also common in pregnant women.
- Copper deficiency in TPN patients presents as anemia and neutropenia.
- Selenium deficiency presents as cardiomyopathy and congestive heart failure (CHF), in conjunction with muscle wasting.
- TPN also can lead to deficiencies in other divalent cations, folate, cobalamin, and fat-soluble vitamins (A, D, E, and K).
- Think of the fat-soluble vitamin deficiencies whenever you are faced with a patient with intestinal or pancreatic problems and resultant malabsorption and steatorrhea.

Vitamin A Deficiency

- *CLASSIC PRESENTATION:* A young to adolescent child who experiences night blindness, eye pain (secondary to corneal erosion), and/or skin changes (dryness, hyperkeratosis).
- Vitamin A deficiency is usually due to dietary deficiency.
- Treatment with Vitamin A may or may not be effective.

Vitamin D Deficiency (Rickets)

- *CLASSIC PRESENTATION:* A poor or debilitated patient, usually a child, who does not eat many vitamin D-fortified foods, particularly dairy products, presents with bone pain and tenderness, as well as muscle weakness. Upon examination, bowing of the legs, disturbances in growth, and swelling of many of the joints may be noted.
- Rare in the U.S. because of fortified foods.
- Treat with Vitamin D.

Vitamin E Deficiency

- *CLASSIC PRESENTATION:* A child with congenital or chronic liver disease presents with a multitude of neurologic abnormalities, especially cerebellar signs.

Vitamin K Deficiency

- *CLASSIC PRESENTATION:* A patient on warfarin therapy presents with bleeding, especially hemarthrosis and large ecchymoses.
- Vitamin K deficiency does not usually present with small petechiae or mucosal bleeding.
- Both the PT and the PTT are prolonged due to decreased synthesis of the vitamin K-dependent clotting factors II, VII, IX, and X.
- Treat with vitamin K, and if applicable, withdrawal of warfarin.

RHEUMATOLOGY

Osteoarthritis

- *CLASSIC PRESENTATION:* An older person presents with deep, aching pain symmetrically involving either large or small joints. Pain is relieved by rest and worsened with exertion. The patient also may have a history of short-duration morning stiffness (less than 30 minutes) and stiffness after inactivity.
- Physical examination is significant for crepitus, painful range of motion, Heberden's nodes (enlargement of DIP joint), and Bouchard's nodes (enlargement of PIP joints)
- Treatment consists of weight loss (for involvement of weight-bearing joints), and isometric exercises. Consider NSAIDs or intra-articular steroid injections.

Acute Gout

- *CLASSIC PRESENTATION:* A middle-aged man with the acute onset of severe pain and signs of inflammation in a small joint, [classically the first (big) toe].
- Diagnosis is by history of gout, or demonstration of needle-shaped crystals that are negatively birefringent in the affected synovial fluid. (with positively birefringent crystals, think of pseudogout instead).
- Treat with NSAIDs, colchicine, intra-articular steroids. Avoid allopurinol and probenecid during acute attacks (use for chronic gout).

Pseudogout (Calcium Pyrophosphate Deposition Disease)

- *CLASSIC PRESENTATION:* An elderly patient with monarticular or pauciarticular arthritis and pain. Clinically indistinguishable from gout, except for its predilection for larger peripheral joints such as the knee.
- Diagnosis is by light microscopy of the synovial fluid. Pseudogout crystals are positively birefringent. Patients also usually have normal uric acid levels.
- Pseudogout is often accompanied by chondrocalcinosis, a characteristic calcification of articular cartilage, visible on x-ray.
- Treat with NSAIDS.

Rheumatoid Arthritis

- *CLASSIC PRESENTATION:* A female patient with bilateral, symmetrical arthritis involving the wrist, MCP, and PIP joints. DIP involvement is rare. Prolonged morning stiffness (>1 hour), and constitutional complaints are common.
- Firm, subcutaneous nodules (rheumatoid nodules) present on extensor surfaces, with soft tissue swelling around joints. Look for anemia of chronic disease, elevated ESR, positive rheumatoid factor.
- Treat with NSAIDs, steroids (usually systemic). Second line agents include sulfasalazine, methotrexate, antimalarial agents, gold, and D-penicillamine.

Systemic Lupus Erythematosus (SLE)

- *CLASSIC PRESENTATION:* A 20- to 40-year-old woman who presents with a "butterfly" rash on her face, weight loss, and generalized fatigue.
- Although the above description is a common way for SLE to present, this is a multisystem disease that may also present in countless other ways.
- More than 80% of SLE is diagnosed in women aged 20 to 40.
- The presence of four out of the following 11 criteria makes the diagnosis of SLE. Use the mnemonic **MD SOAP BRAIN** to remember the criteria:

    Malar rash

    Discoid rash

    Serositis – pleuritis or pericarditis

    Oral ulcers

    Arthritis

    Photosensitivity

    Blood disorders – hemolytic anemia, leukopenia, or thrombocytopenia

    Renal disorders – persistent proteinuria or cellular casts

    Antinuclear antibody positivity

    Immunologic disorders

    Neurologic disorders – seizures or psychosis

- Treatment for SLE is individualized to the features of each particular patient, but may include NSAIDs, antimalarials, corticosteroids, and/or cytotoxic agents.

Less Common Rheumatologic Disorders

- **Ankylosing Spondylitis** - look for young adult males with chronic low back pain and morning stiffness. Associated with HLA B27.
- **Reiter's Syndrome** - look for the simultaneous onset of arthritis, urethritis/cervicitis, dysentery, and/or conjunctivitis/uveitis.
- **Septic Arthritis** – Classically presents with the acute onset of pain, tenderness, and swelling, usually in only one joint. Occasionally there are dermatologic manifestations also. Think *N. gonorrhoeae*, *Staphylococcus* or *Streptococcus*.
- **Scleroderma (Systemic Sclerosis)** - small vessel, skin, and internal organ fibrosis. Look for a patient with skin changes, such as distal skin thickening or Raynaud's phenomenon, along with GI motility disorders (most commonly esophageal). Also may see interstitial lung disease or cardiomyopathy. Raynaud's phenomenon and arthralgias are usually early symptoms. **CREST** syndrome is one form of scleroderma:

    Calcinosis

    Raynaud's phenomenon

    Esophageal dysfunction

    Sclerodactyly

    Telangiectasia

- **Polymyositis** – look for muscle soreness, tenderness, and inflammation with elevated CK.
- **Dermatomyositis** – presents like polymyositis with simultaneous rash. Classically you see erythematous patches diffusely distributed (the distribution is not correlated with that of the myositis).
- **Sjögren's Syndrome (sicca syndrome)** – classically presents with dry eyes and dry mouth, with possible salivary gland enlargement. Antibodies to Ro (SS-A) are common in this idiopathic autoimmune disorder.
- **Polyarteritis Nodosa** – usually presents with constitutional complaints (fever, weight loss, fatigue) and multiorgan ischemic dysfunction (especially renal involvement).

HEMATOLOGY/ONCOLOGY

Anemia
- The first step in searching for a cause of anemia should be to look at the MCV and determine if the anemia is microcytic (below normal MCV), normocytic (normal MCV), or macrocytic (above normal MCV).

Microcytic Anemia
- **Iron deficiency anemia** - common and usually seen in young (menstruating) females or chronic GI bleeders. Look for low ferritin and serum iron, and high total iron binding capacity.
- **Thalassemias** - look for abnormal smear showing poikilocytosis in Asian or Mediterranean populations. Along with iron deficiency, should be high on your differential.
- **Anemia of chronic disease** - often seen with rheumatic disorders (rheumatoid arthritis), serious infections, or carcinomas. Low serum iron and total iron binding capacity are seen, usually with normal ferritin.
- **Sideroblastic anemia** - can be acquired or congenital. The acquired form is often caused by lead, alcohol, or INH therapy. High ferritin and serum iron are seen, with high pulse oxygen saturation. Often there are macrocytic and microcytic cells. Treat with a trial of pyridoxine.

Macrocytic Anemia
- Think about B_{12} and folate deficiency, as discussed above.
- Also seen with increased reticulocyte count (accelerated erythropoiesis), e.g., posthemorrhagic erythropoiesis.
- Drug induced, such as with trimethoprim-sulfamethoxazole, methotrexate, or phenytoin.

Normocytic Anemia

- **Aplastic anemia** - should be considered in patients who present with fatigue, dyspnea (secondary to anemia), easy bruisability, petechiae, mucosal bleeding (secondary to thrombocytopenia) and/or overwhelming infection (due to leukopenia).
- **Posthemorrhagic anemia** - note that this can be either microcytic (secondary to iron deficiency), macrocytic (secondary to increased reticulocyte count) or normocytic.
- **Hemolytic anemia** - often presents acutely with jaundice (or itching and dark urine). Look for positive Coomb's test, increased LDH, and decreased haptoglobin. Often caused by drugs. Heinz bodies are indicative of G6PD deficiency (which is exacerbated by sulfa and quinine drugs in particular).

Sickle Cell Anemia

- *CLASSIC PRESENTATION:* An African-American patient with severe chronic hemolysis with elevated bilirubin, gallstone disease, and/or ulcerations over their lower extremities.
- Patients are functionally asplenic before age 5, with the need for vaccinations against encapsulated organisms (*Pneumococcus*, *Meningococcus*, and *H. influenzae* in particular).
- Sickle cell crises include pain crises, chest crises (a pain crisis with a pulmonary infiltrate), aplastic crises (usually secondary to parvovirus), hyperhemolytic crises, and splenic sequestration crises.

Polycythemia Vera

- *CLASSIC PRESENTATION:* A middle-aged male with a ruddy complexion, severe generalized pruritus (especially after warm showers), splenomegaly, and thrombosis.
- Also associated with increased WBCs and platelets.
- There is excessive production of red blood cells in the bone marrow.
- *BEWARE*! COPD, excessive hypovolemia (diuresis, gastroenteritis, burns), and erythropoietin-producing tumors (hypernephromas) can also cause an increase in hematocrit.

LEUKEMIA AND RELATED DISEASES

Chronic Myelogenous Leukemia (CML)

- *CLASSIC PRESENTATION:* A middle-aged patient with markedly increased WBCs with marked left shift and splenomegaly. May also have fevers, sweats, and fatigue.
- Definitive diagnosis is made by demonstrating the presence of the Philadelphia chromosome (9;22 translocation) on chromosome testing or karyotyping.
- The major cause of death is called a blast crisis, which is progression to a hyperacute phase, similar to AML.

Chronic Lymphocytic Leukemia (CLL)

- *CLASSIC PRESENTATION:* An adult over 50 years old, who is usually asymptomatic at diagnosis, is found on routine laboratory testing to have mature lymphocytosis. Alternatively, patients may present with fatigue, infections, or bleeding.
- Corroborative findings include marrow infiltration by mature lymphocytes, splenomegaly, and lymphadenopathy. Patients may also have anemia, neutropenia, and thrombocytopenia, which account for symptoms at diagnosis.

Acute Myelogenous Leukemia (AML)

- *CLASSIC PRESENTATION:* An adult who presents with fatigue and pallor (due to anemia); fever and infection (due to neutropenia); petechiae, purpura, and epistaxis (due to thrombocytopenia). May also present with infiltrative symptoms (splenomegaly, gum hypertrophy, and bone pain).
- Risk factors for AML include prior radiation therapy or chemotherapy, chemical exposures (benzene), myelodysplasia, myeloproliferative disorders, aplastic anemia, and congenital chromosome disorders (Down's syndrome, Turner's syndrome).
- Average age of onset is 50 years old.
- In the CBC laboratory tests, look for pancytopenia, circulating blast forms (increased WBC not necessary), and elevated uric acid levels. Auer rods in the cytoplasm of blast cells are pathognomonic for AML.
- Can see disseminated intravascular coagulation (DIC) in acute promyelocytic leukemia.

Acute Lymphoblastic Leukemia (ALL)

- See Pediatrics Chapter. Rarely presents in adults.

Lymphoma

- *CLASSIC PRESENTATION:* A patient of any age with persistent enlargement of one or more lymph nodes, in one or more groups of lymph nodes. Patients may experience systemic symptoms such as fevers, chills, and night sweats.
- May be divided into Hodgkin's and Non-Hodgkin's types on basis of pathology. The Reed-Sternberg cell (a multinucleated giant cell) is pathognomonic for Hodgkin's disease.
- Non-Hodgkin's lymphoma may involve extra-nodal organs such as the stomach, lung, and CNS. It is classified as either low, intermediate, or high grade. The presentation varies with the organ affected.
- Hodgkin's lymphoma has a bimodal age distribution, peaking both in patients age 20 to 25 and in patients >55 years old. The median age of onset of non-Hodgkin's lymphoma is 50.
- Staging of Hodgkin's lymphoma:

	Stage
I	Single lymph node group involved
II	Two or more lymph node groups on same side of diaphragm
III	Both sides of the diaphragm involved
IV	Disseminated or extralymphatic disease
	Classification
A	No constitutional symptoms
B	Fever, weight loss, or night sweats

Multiple Myeloma

- *CLASSIC PRESENTATION:* A middle-aged or older patient with bone pain (usually in the back or ribs), pathologic fractures, infection, and/or anemia (which may present as weakness, fatigue, shortness of breath). More common in African Americans.
- Seventy percent of patients present with bone pain. X-ray reveals "punched-out" lytic lesions in bone. The patient may also have hypercalcemia.
- Abnormal plasma cells secrete an overabundance of cell products (either immunoglobulins or subunits).
- Diagnosis is suggested by monoclonal spike on serum or urine electrophoresis.
- A major component of multiple myeloma is renal failure, due to many factors including amyloid deposition in interstitium and renal vasculature, light chain deposition in renal tubules, hypercalcemia, and hyperviscosity of the blood.
- Amyloidosis develops in a minority of patients, and in addition to renal failure, it may lead to CHF and liver disease.

Waldenström's Macroglobulinemia

- *CLASSIC PRESENTATION:* A patient with the symptoms of multiple myeloma, with signs of hyperviscosity including symptoms of visual disturbances and altered mental status. Upon physical examination, adenopathy and hepatosplenomegaly may be seen.
- There is less hypercalcemia than with multiple myeloma.
- In Waldenström's macroglobulinemia, the abnormal cells are B-cells that are differentiating into plasma cells and they secrete IgM.

Coagulopathies

- Petechiae and purpura, along with epistaxis and other mucocutaneous bleeding suggest a platelet disorder or small vessel disorder such as scurvy or paraproteinemia.
- Deep bruises, hematomas, and hemarthroses suggest a disorder of the coagulation pathway.
- Recurrent bleeding since childhood or a positive family history of bleeding disorders suggests an inherited problem.
- A mixed presentation should make you think of von Willebrand's disease, a relatively common disease.

Tumor Markers

- CEA (carcinoembryonic antigen) is increased in colorectal carcinomas, pancreatic carcinoma, and other GI malignancies, as well as some benign conditions (including smoking).
- α-fetoprotein (AFP) is increased in hepatocellular carcinoma, ovarian and testicular germinal carcinomas, and various other benign and malignant conditions.
- Prostate specific antigen (PSA) is elevated in benign prostatic hypertrophy (BPH) as well as prostatic carcinoma. Usually, higher elevations increase the likelihood of carcinoma.
- Urinary vanillylmandelic acid (VMA) is increased in pheochromocytoma, neuroblastoma, and with some medications. False positives may be caused by ingestion of particular foods.
- Urinary 5-hydroxyindoleacetic acid (5-HIAA) and plasma serotonin levels are increased in carcinoid syndrome.
- CA 19-9 is elevated in pancreatic carcinoma.
- CA-125 is elevated in ovarian carcinoma.
- Note that most tumor markers are used to follow the course of a disease with or after therapy, often to watch for recurrences, rather than for diagnostic purposes.

GENETIC DISEASES

Marfan's Syndrome

- *CLASSIC PRESENTATION:* An adolescent with abnormally tall stature, lean body habitus, decreased vision (due to lens dislocation), and aortic root dilatation with or without a dissecting aortic aneurysm.
- Also look for chest wall deformities such as pectus excavatum or carinatum, mitral valve prolapse, and bruising/bleeding manifestations (due to weakened vascular connective tissue).
- Differential diagnosis includes homocystinuria (with similar skeletal and lens changes), and other connective tissue disorders.

Huntington's Disease

- *CLASSIC PRESENTATION:* A 35- to 40-year-old patient who presents with progressive bizarre, choreiform or athetoid movements of limbs and face. Also may present with progressive dementia or emotional changes. Look for a family history of these symptoms.
- Radiographically, you may see atrophy of the caudate nucleus and putamen.
- Caused by an autosomal dominant gene on chromosome 4.

Hemophilia

- *CLASSIC PRESENTATION:* A young male patient presents with signs of deep tissue bleeding such as hematomas, hemarthrosis, or severe prolonged bleeding after surgery or trauma.
- Laboratory test: isolated prolonged PTT, factor VIII (Hemophilia A), or factor IX (Hemophilia B) level is very low.
- Both hemophilia A and B are X-linked recessive traits, and hemophilia B is much less common.

Von Willebrand's Disease

- *CLASSIC PRESENTATION:* A patient with a history of frequent epistaxis, mucosal bleeding, bruising, and prolonged bleeding from wounds. A woman may complain of menorrhagia.
- Autosomal dominant pattern of inheritance of deficiency of von Willebrand's factor.
- Von Willebrand's factor helps platelets adhere to endothelium, stabilizes factor VIII, and enhances platelet aggregation.
- Bleeding time is prolonged and clotting factor VIII levels are reduced. Diagnosis is made by noting platelet dysfunction in the ristocetin cofactor assay.
- Often severe in childhood but generally improves with age.
- Most common inherited hemostatic disorder (about 1/1000 individuals).

Neurofibromatosis

- *CLASSIC PRESENTATION:* A patient of any age with neurofibromas (similar grossly to large skin tags), *"café-au-lait"* spots, hamartomas in the iris (the classic Lisch nodule), or optic gliomas.
- Patients are at risk for astrocytic tumors, compressive neuropathy, pheochromocytoma, and neurofibrosarcoma.
- Autosomal dominant pattern of inheritance.

Familial Hypercholesterolemia

- *CLASSIC PRESENTATION:* (heterozygotes): A patient who has an early MI (in the third or fourth decade), marked hypercholesterolemia (in the 400-500 mg/dL LDL range), and tendon xanthomas on extensor surfaces.

- *CLASSIC PRESENTATION:* (homozygotes) A patient with a much more severe hypercholesterolemia (with an LDL > 1000 mg/dL), cutaneous xanthomas, and history of an MI in the first or second decade of life. Patients often die of early MIs.
- Inheritance is autosomal dominant and results in a mutation of the LDL receptor, leading to increased LDL and total cholesterol levels.

PULMONARY MEDICINE

Pulmonary Function Tests (PFTs)
- Obstructive lung disease (asthma, COPD) - look for a decreased FEV_1/FVC ratio (less than 70%), and increased lung volumes (hyperinflation).
- Restrictive lung disease (pulmonary fibrosis, kyphoscoliosis, chest wall paralysis) - look for a normal to increased FEV_1/FVC ratio and decreased lung volumes.
- Parenchymal lung disease - look for a decreased D_{LCO}, but with hemorrhage or congestion there may be an increased D_{LCO}.

Chronic Obstructive Pulmonary Disease (COPD)
Emphysematous type
- *CLASSIC PRESENTATION:* A patient over 60 years old, usually with an extensive smoking history, presents with progressive exertional dyspnea, weight loss, and little or no cough or expectoration.
- PFTs show little or no response to bronchodilators, and hypocapnia.
- Chest x-ray shows increased lung volumes, hyperlucency, and a flattened diaphragm.

Chronic Bronchitic type
- *CLASSIC PRESENTATION:* A younger smoker with chronic cough and expectoration, episodic dyspnea, and weight gain. Also look for signs and symptoms of cor pulmonale (right heart failure).
- PFTs show response to bronchodilators, and hypercapnia.
- Chest x-ray shows thickened bronchial walls and "dirty" lung fields.

Asthma
- *CLASSIC PRESENTATION:* A patient of any age presents with episodic coughing, dyspnea, chest tightness, and expiratory wheezing.
- Symptoms may be provoked by allergies, preceding URI, exercise, or no discernable etiology.
- Status asthmaticus is asthma that is so severe that it puts the patient at risk for ventilatory failure, and does not respond to appropriate treatment. Patients can die and may need to be intubated.

- Treat with anti-inflammatory drugs such as cromolyn sodium or steroids for long term maintenance. Use bronchodilators such as methylxanthines, β-agonists, or anticholinergics for mild to moderate acute exacerbations. For moderate to severe acute exacerbations, systemic steroid therapy is indicated.

Acute Respiratory Distress Syndrome (ARDS)

- *CLASSIC PRESENTATION:* A patient with chronic lung disease and/or an acute pulmonary insult presents with progressive dyspnea and hypoxia requiring intubation and ventilatory support. Patients may present up to 48 hours after the insult. Physical findings are usually limited to bilateral rales. Chest x-ray shows bilateral "fluffy" infiltrates.
- ARDS is acute hypoxic, hypocapnic respiratory failure caused by diffuse pulmonary capillary leakage resulting in the loss of lung compliance, dyspnea, and hypoxia.
- ARDS can be initiated by many insults, including shock, sepsis, aspiration, DIC, trauma, transfusion, pancreatitis, smoke inhalation, and heroin overdose.
- Management is with intubation, oxygen, and positive end-expiratory pressure ventilation (PEEP). Prognosis is poor.

Pulmonary Embolus

- *CLASSIC PRESENTATION:* A bedridden or otherwise immobile patient presents with the sudden onset of dyspnea at rest and chest pain (usually pleuritic). May also present with syncope and hemoptysis. Pulmonary embolus usually follows prolonged bedrest or a long airline trip, an operative procedure (hip replacement is classic), or a hypercoaguable state (cancer).
- Physical examination shows dullness to percussion and decreased breath sounds. Lower extremities may show tender cord, unilateral edema, or positive Homans' sign.
- Arterial blood gas reveals a widened A-a gradient.
- The gold standard for diagnosis is pulmonary angiography. However, work-up often begins with lower extremity doppler/duplex and a lung ventilation-perfusion (V/Q) scan. Spiral CT of the lungs is also highly accurate.
- Treatment is with heparin, followed by PO warfarin for 4 to 6 months. Occasionally, an IVC filter is placed, usually in patients in whom anticoagulation is contraindicated, or has failed.

Spontaneous Pneumothorax

- *CLASSIC PRESENTATION:* A young, tall, thin male presents with the sudden onset of acute dyspnea and pleuritic chest pain.
- Chest x-ray reveals decreased lung markings in the affected area.
- Treatment involves immediate decompression of the pneumothorax, usually by placement of a chest tube.

Pleural Effusion

- *CLASSIC PRESENTATION:* A patient presents with the gradual onset of dyspnea, pleuritic chest pain, and/or a pericardial friction rub. Physical examination reveals dullness to percussion and decreased breath sounds over the affected lung fields. Chest x-ray shows blunting of the costophrenic angle.
- Transudates contain low total protein, low cell count, and low fluid:serum protein ratios. Etiologies include edematous states such as CHF, nephrotic syndrome, and cirrhosis.
- Exudates contain high total protein, high fluid:serum protein ratios, and variable cell counts. Etiologies include malignancy, inflammatory causes, and trauma.

Sarcoidosis

- *CLASSIC PRESENTATION:* A middle-aged African-American female presents with fatigue, dyspnea on exertion, and a nonproductive cough. She may also present with rashes including erythema nodosum, hepatosplenomegaly, uveitis, arthritis, and other symptoms of systemic involvement. Clinical presentation varies greatly.
- Chest x-ray shows bilateral thoracic lymphadenopathy, as well as possible interstitial infiltrate/fibrosis in advanced stages.
- This is a systemic, noncaseating granulomatous disease. There is lung involvement in 90% of cases.
- Angiotensin-converting enzyme (ACE) levels can be elevated, but this is not very sensitive or specific for sarcoidosis.
- Systemic involvement may include uveitis, various skin lesions, arthritis, Bell's palsy and other cranial nerve palsies, hypercalcemia, and cardiomyopathy.
- Treatment with steroids in some patients.

Obstructive Sleep Apnea

- *CLASSIC PRESENTATION:* An obese male patient with a history of loud snoring, presenting with daytime somnolence, personality changes, or slowed mentation. This may present as recurrent automobile or industrial accidents.
- Complicated by cardiac arrhythmias, pulmonary hypertension, and/or cor pulmonale.
- Treated with weight reduction, continuous positive airway pressure (CPAP), or tracheostomy.

PULMONARY-RENAL SYNDROMES

Goodpasture's Syndrome

- *CLASSIC PRESENTATION:* A patient presents with hemoptysis and dyspnea, often preceded by URI symptoms.

- This is a progressive autoimmune syndrome causing pulmonary hemorrhage and glomerulonephritis progressing to renal failure.
- Look for bilateral alveolar infiltrates on chest x-ray. Definitive diagnosis by demonstrating anti-glomerular basement membrane (anti-GBM) antibodies.

Wegener's Granulomatosis

- *CLASSIC PRESENTATION:* A patient with more systemic involvement than Goodpasture's syndrome, although a similar pulmonary presentation is common.
- This is a systemic vasculitis causing granulomatous inflammation and necrosis of many organs.
- Diagnosed by upper and lower respiratory tract involvement, glomerulonephritis, and detection of circulating antineutrophilic cytoplasmic antibody (c-ANCA).

INFECTIOUS DISEASES

Tuberculosis

- *CLASSIC PRESENTATION:* A homeless patient or new immigrant from a country where tuberculosis infection is prevalent presents with constitutional symptoms such as weight loss, fever, and drenching night sweats, in addition to pulmonary symptomatology, such as a cough with scanty, nonpurulent sputum that may, however, be blood-streaked.
- On chest x-ray primary tuberculosis consists of a Gohn's complex, referring to a calcified hilar lymph node in addition to a calcified peripheral lung lesion.
- Radiographic manifestations of reactivation tuberculosis are very variable, and usually present in the apical lung fields. Classically, there is prominent hilar lymph node enlargement, and apical cavitations on chest x-ray.
- Disseminated tuberculosis may present with a miliary pattern on chest x-ray.
- Extrapulmonary tuberculosis is relatively common. Common sites affected include:
    1. Serosa (pleura, pericardium, and peritoneum) which usually present with an effusion.
    2. Cervical lymph nodes (referred to as scrofula).
    3. Skeletal system (tuberculous disease of the spine is called Pott's disease).
    4. Renal (presenting with microscopic pyuria and hematuria in the face of a sterile culture).
    5. Adrenal.
    6. Miliary tuberculosis refers to a wide, hematogenous dissemination of the tubercle bacilli.
- When is a PPD test considered positive?
    1. >5 mm in HIV-positive and immunocompromised patients

2.   >10 mm in otherwise sick patients, health care workers, high-risk populations
3.   >15 mm in healthy persons

- Chemoprophylaxis with isoniazid (6 months to 1 year) is considered in PPD-positive patients without symptoms and with negative chest films.
- The major considerations in isoniazid prophylaxis are hepatitis (which is age related), age (usually patients under 35 are treated prophylactically, while after that time, the rate of hepatitis MAY become unacceptable), compliance (incomplete compliance can lead to resistant organisms), and vitamin B deficiency (pyridoxine [B$_6$] is usually given concurrently).
- Patients with symptoms, positive acid-fast cultures, and/or positive chest films are usually placed on multi-drug therapy.
- The combination of drugs chosen usually depends on the prevalence of resistant tuberculosis in the community, and on specific antibiotic sensitivity results if they are available.
- Drugs used include isoniazid, rifampin, ethambutol, and pyrazinamide.

Pneumonia
Classical Bacterial Pneumonia
- *CLASSIC PRESENTATION:* A patient presents with shaking chills, fever, pleuritic chest pain, and a productive cough with purulent or rusty sputum. Usually, a recent history of a preceding URI or a prodrome of headache, malaise, and myalgias can be elicited.
- Chest x-ray manifestations include a pulmonary infiltrate, usually confined to one lobe.
- The most common pathogen in adults is *Streptococcus pneumoniae*, or pneumococcus, which is a Gram-positive coccus that usually is found in pairs or short chains.
- COPD patients and smokers are especially prone to develop pneumonia from *Moraxella catarrhalis*. Consider *Klebsiella* in alcoholics.
- Consider *S. aureus* and *Pseudomonas* in hospitalized patients, or those living in nursing homes.
- Treat classic community-acquired lobar pneumonia with a third-generation cephalosporin or a β-lactam/β-lactamase inhibitor such as ampicillin/sulbactam.
- If *Pseudomonas* is a suspected organism, use an appropriate antibiotic such as ceftazidime.

Atypical Pneumonia
- *CLASSIC PRESENTATION:* A patient less than 40 years old who has experienced a prominent flu-like prodrome of fever, sore throat, headaches, myalgias and malaise before the onset of a nonproductive hacking cough and substernal chest pain. In contrast to bacterial pneumonia, purulent sputum and pleuritic chest pain are uncommon.

- Chest radiograph classically shows a diffuse, interstitial pattern without consolidations or infiltrates.

- The most common etiologic agent is *Mycoplasma pneumoniae* (a diagnosis that is often supported by the serologic presence of cold agglutinins). Other causes include *Chlamydia pneumoniae*, and many other viruses.

- Legionnaire's disease (caused by *Legionella pneumophila*) is additionally characterized by diarrhea, abdominal pain, elevated liver enzymes, and relative bradycardia.

- *Pneumocystis carinii* pneumonia (PCP) should be considered in any patient at risk for HIV.

- Treat atypical pneumonia with erythromycin. If PCP is high on your differential, treat with trimethoprim-sulfamethoxazole also.

Aspiration Pneumonia

- *CLASSIC PRESENTATION:* A bedridden patient, or an alcoholic, develops a productive cough with foul-smelling sputum, fevers, and dyspnea.

- Chest x-ray may show a lobar or cavitary pattern, classically in the right middle lobe.

- The most common etiologic agent of a community-acquired aspiration pneumonia is a Gram-negative anaerobe. If the pneumonia is hospital-acquired, consider *S. aureus* and Gram-negative bacteria.

- Treat a community-acquired aspiration pneumonia with cefotetan or clindamycin to cover anaerobes. Appropriate antibiotics should be added if hospital-acquired organisms are suspected.

Human Immunodeficiency Virus (HIV)/Acquired Immunodeficiency Syndrome (AIDS)

- *CLASSIC PRESENTATION:* Patients who are HIV-positive but do not have AIDS are usually asymptomatic except for a short viral prodrome within a few weeks to months after exposure to HIV, which may be characterized by headaches, fevers, adenopathy, and rashes which resolve on their own within days to weeks. Patients with AIDS have evidence of HIV infection, fewer than 200 CD4 cells/μL of blood, and usually present with a specific opportunistic infection or malignancy.

- HIV is a retrovirus that is transmitted from person to person by sexual activity, sharing of blood (transfusion or IV drug abuse), or a transplacental mechanism. IV drug abuse and heterosexual activity account for the most recent rises in new infections, especially among women.

- Diagnosis is by a blood test in which HIV-antibody presence is determined by ELISA, with confirmation of the presence of viral proteins by Western blot.

- HIV patients in therapy are followed by monitoring their clinical symptoms, their CD4 counts, and the viral load by PCR.

- Opportunistic infections that are commonly the presenting signs of AIDS include *Pneumocystis carinii* pneumonia, toxoplasmosis, histoplasmosis, cryptococcal meningitis, cytomegalovirus infection, herpes simplex virus infection, miliary tuberculosis, *Mycobacterium avium* infection, and candidiasis.

- Malignancies that commonly develop in AIDS patients include Kaposi's sarcoma and lymphomas.
- Treatment for HIV-positive patients includes the use of antiretroviral agents such as nucleoside analog reverse transcriptase inhibitors (e.g., AZT, ddI, 3TC), protease inhibitors (e.g., indinavir, ritonavir, saquinavir), and nonnucleoside reverse transcriptase inhibitors (e.g., nevirapine, delavirdine).
- Patients with CD4 counts less than 200 cells/μL should receive prophylaxis against *Pneumocystis carinii* pneumonia with trimethoprim-sulfamethoxazole.

NEPHROLOGY

Nephrolithiasis
- *CLASSIC PRESENTATION:* A patient presents with the sudden onset of flank pain, often radiating to the inguinal ligament or urogenital structures, hematuria, nausea, vomiting, and urinary frequency. He may also have dysuria, and frequently has a past history of kidney stones.
- The vast majority of renal stones are radio-opaque. Exceptions are uric acid stones.
- Treatment varies with the type of stone. Acutely, hydrate to increase urine output, and provide adequate pain control.

Urinary Tract Infection (UTI)
- *CLASSIC PRESENTATION:* for lower UTI: A patient with urinary frequency, dysuria, and malodorous or cloudy urine. Hematuria may be present. There may be suprapubic tenderness on physical examination.
- *CLASSIC PRESENTATION:* for upper UTI: A patient with the above symptoms plus flank pain, fever, and malaise. May also have nausea and vomiting.
- On a clean catch specimen, $>10^5$ colonies/ml is indicative of a UTI. For a catheter specimen, $>10^4$ colonies/ml is sufficient. For a specimen obtained through a suprapubic tube, 1 colony/ml is sufficient to diagnose an infection.
- The most common organisms are *E. coli, S. saprophyticus, Klebsiella,* and *P. mirabilis* (suspect this organism if you see a high urinary ph).
- Treatment of uncomplicated cystitis can be with trimethoprim-sulfamethoxazole, fluoroquinolones, sulfonamides, or amoxicillin. Uncomplicated pyelonephritis may be treated with an IV third generation cephalosporin or ampicillin and gentamicin in severely ill patients.
- Treatment of recurrent cystitis is often prophylaxis with a sulfonamide, trimethoprim-sulfamethoxazole, or a fluoroquinolone.

Acute Renal Failure

- *CLASSIC PRESENTATION:* A patient presents with a rapid increase in BUN and creatinine. Urine output is variable, but patients are often oliguric (<400 ml of urine output/day).
- Etiologies:
    1. Prerenal – decreased renal perfusion, either by volume depletion, decreased cardiac output, or a decrease in intravascular volume. The BUN:creatinine ratio is >20:1 and fractional excretion of sodium is <1.
    2. Postrenal – obstruction of the urinary tract, commonly by an enlarged prostate, gynecologic disease, or bilateral renal stones. On ultrasound there is hydronephrosis. The BUN:creatinine ratio is >20:1, and the fractional excretion of sodium is <1.
    3. Intrinsic – caused by disease of the kidney itself. There may be glomerular disease, vascular disease (renal artery or vein thrombosis or embolism, vasculitis, etc.), acute interstitial nephritis, or acute tubular necrosis. The BUN:creatinine ratio is usually <20:1 and the fractional secretion of sodium is >1.
- Complications of acute renal failure include fluid and electrolyte imbalances, infection, and uremia. Uremia can cause pericarditis, anemia, bleeding disorders, GI disturbances, and CNS disorders.
- Treatment includes IV diuretics, matching fluid and salt intake and output, limiting potassium intake, decreasing protein intake, and aggressive treatment of infection. Dialysis is used in refractory cases.

Indications for Urgent Dialysis

- Remember the mnemonic **AEIOU**:

    Acidosis

    Electrolytes abnormal – specifically, hyperkalemia

    Ingestions – theophylline, lithium, methanol, aspirin

    Overload of fluid – failed high dose furosemide

    Uremia – severe, with pericarditis or altered mental status

Chronic Renal Failure

- *CLASSIC PRESENTATION:* A patient with a history of renal disease with a gradually decreasing glomerular filtration rate, increasing creatinine, hyperkalemia, and hypocalcemia. On ultrasound the kidneys appear small and shrunken.
- Kidneys have decreased endocrine function (decreased erythropoietin with decreased RBC production), decreased enzymatic activity (decreased ammonia synthesis and activation of vitamin D), decreased insulin metabolism (more susceptible to hypoglycemia), and decreased gastrin metabolism (increase in peptic ulceration).

- Serum creatinine level is used to quantify glomerular impairment, with BUN being less precise.
- Etiologies include a few reversible causes (early obstruction, analgesic abuse), diabetes mellitus, hypertension, glomerulonephritis, interstitial and tubular nephritis, hypercalciuria, uric acid nephropathy, and polycystic kidney disease.
- A major complication is uremic syndrome, in which patients display signs of wasting, skin purpura and excoriations, pruritus, nausea, vomiting, and decreased appetite. They also may develop neurologic symptoms, pericarditis and cardiovascular impairment, anemia, and gastrointestinal problems.
- Initial management includes a renal ultrasound to rule out obstruction, and a urinalysis, urine culture, and chemistry panels for further evaluation.
- Diet should be changed to restrict protein, potassium, and phosphate intake. However, when renal function declines by 80% to 90%, chronic renal failure can no longer be controlled with diet and dialysis is indicated.
- Renal transplant can also be considered.

Polycystic Kidney Disease
- *CLASSIC PRESENTATION*: A young adult presents with an enlarging flank mass, abdominal pain, and slowly progressive renal failure.
- This is a genetic disease with an autosomal dominant inheritance pattern. End-stage renal disease develops almost uniformly.
- Polycystic kidney disease is associated with hepatic cysts and intracerebral berry aneurysms.

Alport's Syndrome
- *CLASSIC PRESENTATION*: A patient with progressive renal failure and high frequency hearing loss. Renal failure is indicated by hematuria, RBC casts, proteinuria, and pyuria.
- No effective treatment is currently available.

Acute Glomerulonephritis
- *CLASSIC PRESENTATION*: A patient with gross hematuria, proteinuria, azotemia, and diastolic hypertension.
- Common causes include: postinfectious glomerulonephritis (most commonly 6 to 10 days after streptococcal pharyngitis), autoimmune disease (SLE, IgA nephropathy), and serum sickness.
- One third to one half of cases have progressive deterioration in renal function. Treatment for all forms is supportive.
- Rapidly progressive forms characterized pathologically by "crescent" formation.

Acute Interstitial Nephritis

- *CLASSIC PRESENTATION:* A patient with acute renal failure who also has symptoms of fevers and a rash. CBC reveals eosinophilia.
- Most common cause is drugs, particularly β-lactam antibiotics, NSAIDs, and diuretics. May also be caused by systemic diseases (sarcoidosis, Sjögren's syndrome, lymphoma) and systemic infections (syphilis, toxoplasmosis, viruses), with which symptoms besides renal failure are not usually present.

Acute Tubular Necrosis

- *CLASSIC PRESENTATION:* A patient with acute renal failure following an episode of renal ischemia (due to shock, trauma, hypoxia or sepsis), or exposure to nephrotoxins.
- Nephrotoxins include heavy metals, ethylene glycol, contrast media, and aminoglycosides.
- May also be caused by tumor lysis syndrome or rhabdomyolysis.

Nephrotic Syndrome

- *CLASSIC PRESENTATION:* A patient presents with gradual edema of the entire body (not dependent edema of the legs as in CHF). On routine urinalysis you discover proteinuria (>3.5 g/d). Blood tests reveal hypoalbuminemia and hyperlipidemia.
- A hypercoagulable state makes thromboembolic complications common, so beware of renal vein thrombosis.
- Causes include minimal change disease, the glomerulonephritides, and systemic diseases such as diabetes mellitus and systemic lupus erythematosus.

Renal Cell Carcinoma

- *CLASSIC PRESENTATION:* An older patient with hematuria, an enlarging abdominal mass, flank pain, and weight loss.
- Ultrasound, CT, and an intravenous pyelogram (IVP) may help distinguish this from a transitional cell carcinoma.

Transitional Cell Carcinoma

- *CLASSIC PRESENTATION:* An older patient with hematuria, bladder irritability, and systemic symptoms such as fatigue.
- Associated with tobacco use, occupational carcinogens (dyes, rubber, etc.), schistosomiasis, and phenacetin use.
- May strike anywhere from the renal pelvis to the bladder. IVP and cystoscopy are useful diagnostically.

ELECTROLYTE ABNORMALITIES

Acid-Base Status

- To determine a patient's acid-base status, first look at the pH on the arterial blood gas. Less than 7.35 is acidotic, greater than 7.45 is alkalotic. If the patient is acidotic, determine the anion gap

$$AG = [Na^+] - \{[Cl^-] + [HCO_3^-]\}$$

  If this is increased (normal is 9-12), there is a component of anion-gap metabolic acidosis.
- Next, determine if the CO_2 is increased or decreased. If this is appropriate to the acid-base status (i.e., if it is increased in acidosis, decreased in alkalosis), the primary disturbance is respiratory. If the opposite is true, the primary disturbance is metabolic.

Metabolic Acidosis

- To determine the etiology, first calculate the anion gap:
- Anion gap acidosis (anion gap > 12) is caused by **MUDPILES**:

  Methanol

  Uremia

  Diabetic ketoacidosis

  Paraldehyde

  INH or **I**ron

  Lactic acidosis

  Ethylene glycol

  Salicylates
- Nonanion gap acidosis is commonly caused by renal tubular acidosis and diarrhea.

Metabolic Alkalosis

- To determine the etiology, first determine the urine chloride level.
- Urine chloride of <20 mEq/L will correct with chloride administration. Etiologies include prerenal causes (like CHF), vomiting, and diuretics.
- Urine chloride of >20 mEq/L will not usually correct with chloride administration. Etiologies include Cushing's syndrome and primary hyperaldosteronism.

Hyperkalemia

- *CLASSIC PRESENTATION:* A patient with decreased deep tendon reflexes, weakness/paralysis, or paresthesias. Look for this in patients with chronic renal failure, patients who have received blood transfusions or chemotherapy, or patients in diabetic ketoacidosis.
- EKG changes include peaked T waves and prolonged intervals leading to ventricular fibrillation and eventually asystole.
- Treatment is with calcium gluconate (does not lower serum K), sodium bicarbonate, glucose and insulin, or furosemide.

Hypernatremia

- *CLASSIC PRESENTATION:* A patient with altered mental status, which can progress to seizures. Look for this in nursing home or bed-ridden patients who may not have access to adequate hydration.
- Correct hypernatremia with IV fluids slowly (over 48 hours) to prevent cerebral edema or central pontine myelinolysis.

Hypercalcemia

- *CLASSIC PRESENTATION:* Think "Bones, stones, abdominal groans". A patient with bone pain, kidney stones, abdominal pain, and mental status changes. Look for this especially in patients with malignancy of any type.
- The most common causes are hyperparathyroidism and malignancy (either directly or through PTH-related peptide paraneoplastic syndrome)
- EKG changes show shortened QT interval, with a prolonged PR interval.
- Treatment is with hydration, furosemide, and bisphosphonates.

Hypocalcemia

- *CLASSIC PRESENTATION:* A patient with perioral paresthesias, increased deep tendon reflexes, tetany, cramps, and seizures a few days after a thyroidectomy. Look for facial muscle spasm after tapping the facial nerve (Chvostek's sign) or carpal spasm after occluding the blood flow to the forearm (Trousseau's sign).
- Causes include intestinal bypass surgery, vitamin D deficiency, acute pancreatitis, or thyroidectomy.
- EKG findings include lengthened QT interval (at risk for sudden death!).

GASTROENTEROLOGY

Achalasia

- *CLASSIC PRESENTATION:* A 20- to 40-year-old patient with progressive dysphagia for solids and liquids, accompanied by significant weight loss and chest pain. The patient may also may have nocturnal cough or aspiration pneumonia.

- The diagnosis made by barium swallow, which shows a dilated, flaccid esophagus with beak-like (or "rat's tail") tapering over the lower esophageal sphincter (LES). Manometry shows increased LES pressure and lack of relaxation of the LES.
- Treat with nitrates, β-agonists, calcium channel blockers, or balloon dilation.

Gastritis

- *CLASSIC PRESENTATION:* A patient presents with burning epigastric abdominal pain, nausea, and vomiting. The patient may also have signs of GI bleeding, such as melena or bloody emesis.
- Etiologies include NSAIDs, alcohol, stress (especially induced by illness), and *H. pylori*.
- Test for *H. pylori* infection with a carbon dioxide breath test or serum antibodies.
- Diagnosis made by endoscopy. Treatment is with acid reduction measures (H_2-blockers, H^+/K^+ pump blockers, or mucosal protectants such as sucralfate) and/or antibiotics for *H. pylori* infection.

Malabsorption

- *CLASSIC PRESENTATION:* A patient complains of the passage of greasy, soft, foul smelling stools and significant weight loss. Advanced cases may manifest edema, anemia, coagulopathy, or pathologic fractures.
- Etiologies include pancreatic insufficiency, obstructive or cholestatic liver disease, blind loop syndromes, intrinsic small bowel disease, and extensive small bowel resection.
- Diagnostic work-up should include Sudan black testing for fat in stool, D-xylose tests, and bile acid breath tests.

Celiac Disease

- *CLASSIC PRESENTATION:* A patient presents with symptoms of malabsorption. His symptoms began in childhood, but remitted and reappeared later. May present with iron deficiency anemia that is not associated with GI blood loss.
- This disorder is thought to arise from gluten hypersensitivity.
- Diagnosis is made by small bowel biopsy, which shows flattening of the intestinal villi.
- Treat by elimination of sources of gluten from the diet (wheat, rye, barley, oats).
- Complications include lymphoma or carcinoma (especially esophageal), ulcers, strictures, or skin lesions.

Gastroesophageal Reflux Disease

- *CLASSIC PRESENTATION:* A patient presents with symptoms of heartburn (burning sensation in epigastrium or thoracic area), usually made worse by lying down. Also may present with angina or atypical chest pain.
- Treatment is with acid reduction techniques such as H_2-blockers or antacids.

- Beware of the development of Barrett esophagus, a metaplasia of esophageal squamous epithelium to adenomatous epithelium secondary to reflux. This is a precancerous lesion.

Peptic Ulcer Disease

- *CLASSIC PRESENTATION:* of a duodenal ulcer: A patient who complains of epigastric burning or gnawing pain that occurs approximately 1.5 to 3 hours after eating, which is relieved by food. Pain is usually worse at night, and absent in the morning.
- *CLASSIC PRESENTATION:* of a gastric ulcer: A patient presents with a similar pain syndrome to that for a duodenal ulcer, except for the fact that food may actually precipitate pain.
- Medical treatment for both types of ulcers is with H_2-blockers or antacid, however gastric ulcers are generally harder to treat. Antibiotics should be used if *H. pylori* is suspected.
- Gastric ulcers should be biopsied to rule out gastric carcinoma.

Mesenteric Ischemia (Intestinal Angina)

- *CLASSIC PRESENTATION:* An elderly patient with evidence of other vascular disease (history of a CVA, coronary artery disease, or peripheral vascular disease), who presents with intermittent, crampy, dull, periumbilical pain beginning 15 to 30 minutes after eating and lasting up to several hours. Weight loss is often present secondary to pain-induced anorexia.
- Abdominal films reveal a thumbprinting pattern due to thickened mucosal folds.
- Often relieved by nitrates, which cause vasodilation.

Acute Viral Hepatitis

- *CLASSIC PRESENTATION:* A patient presents with acute or gradual development of signs and symptoms which may include jaundice, nausea, vomiting, malaise, anorexia, and fatigue in the setting of hepatic enlargement or tenderness. Note that jaundice only occurs in about half of the cases.
- Hepatitis A is transmitted through fecal-oral contamination and is not associated with chronic infection or a carrier state. This usually presents acutely.
- Hepatitis B is transmitted parenterally, and chronic disease or a carrier state develops in about 10% of patients. Hepatitis B infection can lead to the development of cirrhosis or hepatomas.
- A favorite examination question is to give a patient's titers (+ or -) for different hepatitis B serologies, and ask what pattern of infection pattern is consistent with (e.g., acute vs. chronic infection). The table below summarizes the different possibilities.

Hepatitis B (HB) Serologies				
Condition	HBsAg	Anti-HBsAb	Anti-HBcAb	HBeAg
Acute HB	+	−	IgM	+
Chronic active HB	+	−	IgG	+
Recovered/latent HB	−	+	IgG	−
After HB vaccination	−	+	−	−

HB = hepatitis B; Ag = antigen; Ab = antibody; s = surface; c = core; e = e

- Hepatitis C is transmitted parenterally and is often associated with hepatitis after transfusion. Chronic hepatitis occurs in 30% to 50% of patients, and many of these go on to develop cirrhosis.
- Hepatitis D is an incomplete virus that is transmitted with the hepatitis B virus.
- Hepatitis E is spread by the fecal-oral route like hepatitis A, and can cause a fulminant hepatitis in pregnant women with a 20% mortality.

Alcoholic Liver Disease
- *CLASSIC PRESENTATION:* Any patient with a significant alcohol history who presents with stigmata of hepatic failure, such as GI bleeding (secondary to gastritis, ulcers, variceal bleeding, or hemorrhoids), jaundice, ascites, palmar erythema, or hepatic encephalopathy (delirium, asterixis).
- Spectrum of disease includes asymptomatic steatohepatitis, acute alcoholic hepatitis (which presents similarly to acute viral hepatitis), and cirrhosis with hepatic failure (as described above).
- Look for increased GGT and AST out of proportion to ALT.

Wilson's Disease (Hepatolenticular Degeneration)
- *CLASSIC PRESENTATION:* A younger than 40-year-old patient with symptoms of hepatic disease along with behavioral, psychiatric, and neurologic (usually Parkinsonian) abnormalities. Classically, slit lamp examination shows a Kayser-Fleischer ring in the cornea.
- Caused by an autosomal recessive deficiency of ceruloplasmin, required for copper transport.

Inflammatory Bowel Disease

- *CLASSIC PRESENTATION:* Commonly, a young patient (age 15 to 30) or an older patient (age 55 to 60) who presents with colicky lower abdominal pain, diarrhea, fever, weight loss, and malaise. Crohn's disease may present with obstruction, while ulcerative colitis is likely to present with bloody diarrhea.
- Crohn's disease is a granulomatous disease that can involve the entire GI tract, from mouth to anus, though the ileum is the most common site of involvement. Pathologically it is characterized by transmural inflammation, ulcerations, and stricture formation. Affected areas may be interspersed between normal areas.
- Ulcerative colitis is confined to the colon, and consists of a contiguous area of inflammation, stretching proximally from the rectum. Inflammation is classically confined to the mucosa, without granuloma or ulcer formation. Radiographically, there is a loss of haustral markings, giving the colon a "lead pipe" appearance. Careful and regular screening should be performed, as ulcerative colitis can often progress to colon carcinoma.
- Extraintestinal manifestations of inflammatory bowel disease include: dermatologic changes (erythema nodosum, pyoderma gangrenosum, aphthous stomatitis), polyarthritis, uveitis, and biliary abnormalities (cholelithiasis, sclerosing cholangitis).

Upper GI Bleeding

- Defined as bleeding from a source above the ligament of Treitz.
- Patients usually present with bloody emesis and/or melena (black, tarry stools), however they may also present with bright red blood in their stool.
- The most common causes include peptic ulcer disease, gastritis, esophageal varices, and an esophageal mucosal tear (Mallory-Weiss tear from excessive vomiting).

Lower GI Bleeding

- Defined as bleeding from a source below the ligament of Treitz.
- Patients usually present with bright red blood in their stool, although they may occasionally have melena. They do not present with bloody emesis.
- The most common causes include hemorrhoids, diverticulosis, angiodysplasia (A-V malformations), inflammatory bowel disease, ischemic colitis, proctitis, and colon cancer.

Carcinoid Syndrome

- *CLASSIC PRESENTATION:* A patient who presents with periodic flushing, intractable diarrhea, and valvular heart disease.
- Carcinoid tumors are neuroendocrine tumors that arise most commonly from the enterochromaffin cells of the GI tract, but can occur throughout the body.
- Effects are due to serotonin secretion by the tumor. Note that GI carcinoid tumors will only present with carcinoid syndrome after the tumor has metastasized to the liver, otherwise the liver will remove the serotonin via first-pass metabolism.

- Diagnosis is made by urinary 5-HIAA levels and serum serotonin levels.

ENDOCRINOLOGY

Pituitary Adenoma
- *CLASSIC PRESENTATION:* A patient complains of the gradual onset of headaches and visual loss starting in superior temporal quadrants that progresses to bitemporal hemianopia. May present with hormonal excess such as Cushing's syndrome, acromegaly, galactorrhea, or amenorrhea.
- Microadenomas are very common. Most present with galactorrhea and/or amenorrhea secondary to prolactin excess. Bromocriptine or phenothiazines may be helpful for these.

Acromegaly
- *CLASSIC PRESENTATION:* An adult patient with increasing ring, glove, shoe, and/or hat sizes. Also has coarsening of facial features.
- This is caused by increased growth hormone secretion after closure of the epiphyseal plates (as an adult). If there is increased growth hormone secretion before fusion of the epiphyseal plates (as a child), gigantism occurs.
- Also present are glucose intolerance and hyperphosphatemia.
- In the vast majority of cases, acromegaly is due to a pituitary adenoma.

Diabetes Insipidus (DI)
- *CLASSIC PRESENTATION:* A patient who complains of severe polyuria and thirst (polydipsia). May follow damage or trauma to the pituitary area.
- The urine osmolality is low (<200 mOsm/kg, specific gravity <1.005), with slightly elevated serum osmolality (helps to differentiate from psychogenic polydipsia, with low serum osmolality).
- Central DI is caused by a decrease in antidiuretic hormone (ADH) secretion by the neurohypophysis, while nephrogenic DI is caused by a lack of renal response to ADH (ADH levels are increased or normal).
- Central DI responds to ADH administration with a rise in urine osmolality, while nephrogenic DI does not.
- A classic on examinations is to present a table such as shown below and to ask you which set of values is consistent with central DI, nephrogenic DI, primary polydipsia, and control (normal).

Serum and Urine Osmolality in Polyuric States				
Condition	Serum osmolality	Urine osmolality	Urine osmolality with dehydration	Urine osmolality after ADH challenge
Normal	Normal	50-1400 mosm/kg	Increased	Increased
Primary polydipsia	Low/normal	Low[2]	Increased	Unchanged[1]
Central diabetes insipidus	High	Low[2]	Unchanged	Increased
Nephrogenic diabetes insipidus	High	Low	Unchanged	Unchanged

[1]Massive free water clearance causes a washout of the renal medullary concentration gradient, and hence impairs renal responsiveness to ADH.

[2]This refers to a urine that is inappropriately dilute in the setting of a high serum osmolality (when one would expect maximally concentrated urine). Beware, because the urine osmolality is usually within the normal range.

Syndrome of Inappropriate ADH Release (SIADH)

- *CLASSIC PRESENTATION:* A patient with established CNS or pulmonary disease presents with symptoms of hyponatremia (confusion, headaches). Hyponatremia is almost invariably present, but urinary sodium excretion is high (>20 mEq/L).
- Can be either a central or paraneoplastic origin of excess ADH secretion.
- Treatment is with fluid restriction or demeclocycline.

Hyperthyroidism

- *CLASSIC PRESENTATION:* A female 20 to 50 years old presents with heat intolerance, weight loss, tachycardia or palpitations, and diarrhea. Look for tremor and wide pulse pressure on physical examination.
- Most commonly due to Graves' disease (positive thyroid stimulating antibodies) which also manifests with exophthalmos and pretibial myxedema.
- Treat with antithyroid drugs, subtotal thyroidectomy, or radioactive iodine. β-blockers ful in thyroid storm (sudden exacerbation of symptoms).

Hypothyroidism
- *CLASSIC PRESENTATION:* A female patient with fatigue, lethargy, cold intolerance, and constipation. A puffy appearance is noted on physical examination.
- Most common etiology is chronic thyroiditis (Hashimoto's thyroiditis). Can also occur after treatment of hyperthyroidism. Iodine deficiency is a common cause in some areas of the world, but is rare in the U.S.
- Myxedema coma may result in severe cases and is a life-threatening manifestation of hypothyroidism. This can present with hypothermia, hypoglycemia, and shock as well as the altered mental status and lethargy.
- Treatment is with L-thyroxine. It should be given IV in cases of myxedema coma.

Thyroid Carcinoma
- *CLASSIC PRESENTATION:* An asymptomatic patient is found to have a single, solid, nontender thyroid mass on physical examination. There is variable uptake of radioactive iodine by the mass, but cancers are more often described as "cold" nodules (due to reduced iodine uptake). Most patients are euthyroid.
- Most common is papillary CA, followed by follicular CA, medullary CA, and anaplastic CA.
- Follicular CA can not be diagnosed by fine-needle aspiration, and information on tissue architecture is necessary for diagnosis.
- Medullary CA secretes calcitonin and can be found as part of the multiple endocrine neoplasia II syndrome (see below).
- Anaplastic CA has an extremely poor prognosis, and is always considered stage 4 at the time of diagnosis.

Multiple Endocrine Neoplasia (MEN Syndromes)
- Type I *CLASSIC PRESENTATION:* A patient with hypercalcemia (parathyroid hyperplasia), intractable gastric ulcers (Zollinger-Ellison syndrome), and visual field defects (pituitary adenoma). Think of the three P's:

    Pancreas

    Pituitary

    Parathyroid

- Type IIA consists of medullary thyroid CA, pheochromocytoma, and parathyroid hyperplasia.
- Type IIB consists of mucosal neuromas, medullary thyroid CA, and pheochromocytoma. Patients usually have a marfanoid body habitus.

Cushing's Syndrome

- *CLASSIC PRESENTATION:* A patient can present with any of a spectrum of symptoms including central obesity (manifesting as moon-like facies and a dorsal fat pad), muscle wasting or weakness, excessive bruisability, and purple striae on the skin. Objective findings include hypertension, hyperglycemia (due to glucose intolerance), and osteoporosis.
- This syndrome is caused by an excess of glucocorticoids.
- The most common cause is iatrogenic (exogenous steroid administration). Cushing's disease, which is pituitary hypersecretion of ACTH leading to adrenal hyperplasia, is the most common noniatrogenic cause.
- Other causes include adrenal adenomas and paraneoplastic syndromes (classically small cell lung CA).
- Work-up of spontaneous Cushing's syndrome should include low-dose and high-dose dexamethasone administration. Normal individuals will suppress cortisol synthesis with even low doses of dexamethasone. Individuals with Cushing's disease will require high doses of dexamethasone to suppress cortisol synthesis. Individuals with paraneoplastic ACTH secretion will not suppress cortisol synthesis even with high doses of dexamethasone.
- Also remember that ACTH hypersecretion causes skin hyperpigmentation, a potentially important diagnostic clue.

Addison's Disease (Primary Adrenal Insufficiency)

- *CLASSIC PRESENTATION:* A patient in whom systemic symptoms predominate, including anorexia, nausea, vomiting, hypotension, and hypoglycemia. Other findings include hyponatremia and hyperkalemia secondary to hypoaldosteronism in primary adrenal insufficiency. Sudden adrenal insufficiency can lead to fever, abdominal pain, and life-threatening vascular collapse.
- Atrophy of the adrenal glands is the most common cause. Other causes include extrapulmonary tuberculosis, and poststeroid therapy adrenal insufficiency (which may manifest in stressful situations for 12 to 18 months after discontinuing steroid therapy).
- Work-up of adrenal insufficiency begins with an ACTH challenge. Lack of cortisol response to an ACTH challenge indicates primary adrenal insufficiency.
- Also indicative of primary insufficiency is ACTH-induced hyperpigmentation, and hypoaldosteronism. Sufficient cortisol response to ACTH challenge may indicate secondary adrenal insufficiency.

Diabetes Mellitus (DM)

- *CLASSIC PRESENTATION:* Type I DM: A young (<20-year-old), thin patient with polyuria and polydipsia. Alternatively, type I DM may initially present as diabetic ketoacidosis (DKA). This classically presents with a hypotensive patient in a coma with an acetone odor on the breath.

- Mainstays of management of DKA include insulin therapy, aggressive hydration, electrolyte (especially potassium) monitoring and repletion, and a search for a precipitating factor (usually an infection). Type I diabetics must receive insulin therapy.
- *CLASSIC PRESENTATION:* Type II DM: A middle-aged, obese patient with polyuria, polydipsia, and a family history of type II DM.
- Type II diabetics can be managed with diet and exercise regimens, oral hypoglycemic drugs, or insulin therapy. They are not prone to develop DKA, however they may develop hyperosmolar nonketotic coma. This occurs mainly in elderly patients, and has a high mortality rate. Patients have a marked hyperglycemia, but no ketosis.
- Complications of both types of DM include atherosclerosis of large vessels, retinopathy, nephropathy, neuropathy (often paresthesias or numbness in a "stocking-glove" distribution), gastroparesis, orthostatic hypotension, and microvascular angiopathy. The latter often leads to chronic ulcers in the feet, osteomyelitis, and eventual amputation. All of these complications are less frequent with better control of blood glucose levels.

TOXICOLOGY

Anticholinergic Toxicity
- *CLASSIC PRESENTATION:* A patient presents with blurred vision, palpitations or a rapid heartbeat, flushed but dry skin, and urinary retention. Upon physical examination you notice mydriasis.
- Anticholinergic toxicity can be caused by tricyclic antidepressants, phenothiazines, and antihistamines, as well as various other medications and illicit drugs with anticholinergic activity.
- Therapy is usually supportive. Physostigmine may be useful in severe cases with seizures or cardiac arrhythmias.

Tricyclic Antidepressant Toxicity
- *CLASSIC PRESENTATION:* A patient presents with anticholinergic signs as described above, PLUS neurologic signs such as altered mental status, ataxia, or hyperreflexia. Severe poisoning can present with coma, hypotension, and respiratory depression.
- EKG findings include prolonged PR, QRS, and QT intervals, and frequent PVCs.
- Management is supportive with cardiovascular monitoring. Gastric lavage and activated charcoal may be useful acutely. Sodium bicarbonate therapy may be used in the treatment of resultant cardiac arrhythmias.

Alcohol Poisonings

- *CLASSIC PRESENTATION:* of methanol poisoning: A similar picture to ethanol intoxication, but patient also complains of significant GI distress with nausea and vomiting. Classically, the patient also complains of visual changes, often described as "looking at a snowstorm."
- *CLASSIC PRESENTATION:* of ethylene glycol poisoning: A patient may present similar to ethanol poisoning, but later develops cardiovascular effects such as tachycardia or CHF. One to three days post ingestion, the patient may complain of costovertebral angle (CVA) tenderness and flank pain. This may be a precursor to acute tubular necrosis and acute renal failure.
- For both types, look for an increased anion gap metabolic acidosis, and an increased osmolal gap. Osmolal gap is defined as (measured serum osmoles)-(calculated serum osmoles). Serum osmoles are calculated as

$$2[Na^+] + [BUN]/2.8 + [glucose]/18$$

- Treatment is with ethanol administration (IV or PO), or dialysis.

Aspirin Toxicity

- *CLASSIC PRESENTATION:* A patient who complains of gastrointestinal symptoms (including vomiting, abdominal pain, evidence of an upper GI bleed), tinnitus and mental status changes (which may progress to seizures). The patient may exhibit either increased or decreased (with severe toxicity) respiratory rate.
- Classically, the arterial blood gas analysis reveals a mixed respiratory alkalosis and metabolic acidosis.
- The patient may manifest signs of pulmonary and cerebral edema. In some cases, cerebral edema is the proximate cause of death.
- Treatment is with charcoal and dialysis if indicated. Alkalinization of the patient's urine can aid excretion.

Acetaminophen Toxicity

- *CLASSIC PRESENTATION:* Patients who acutely ingest toxic quantities of acetaminophen may present in any of four stages:
  - Stage I (7 to 14 hours after ingestion): nausea and vomiting, anorexia, diaphoresis.
  - Stage II (24 to 48 hours after ingestion): symptoms above improve, but the patient may develop right upper quadrant pain and tenderness, an increased liver size, and marked elevation of hepatic transaminases.
  - Stage III (72 to 96 hours after ingestion): this occurs in a minority of patients, but is marked by hepatic necrosis, and manifests clinically as coagulopathy, jaundice, and hypoglycemia. There is a further rise in transaminase levels.

- Stage IV (7 to 8 days after ingestion): this is the recovery phase. However, some patients progress to death from fulminant hepatic failure.
- Treatment, if caught early, is charcoal administration and N-acetylcysteine, which can lessen hepatic injury.

Digitalis Toxicity

- *CLASSIC PRESENTATION:* of acute digitalis toxicity: A patient with nausea, vomiting, and altered mental status. EKG will show supraventricular tachyarrhythmias and A-V block. Laboratory results show hyperkalemia.
- *CLASSIC PRESENTATION:* of chronic digitalis toxicity: An elderly patient, usually on diuretics as well, who presents with nausea, vomiting, and mental status changes, but also reports characteristic visual changes (yellow halos around objects). EKG shows frequent PVCs, and A-V block. Laboratory shows hypokalemia.
- Renal insufficiency, hepatic dysfunction, hypothyroidism, and COPD can all lead to an inadvertent rise in digitalis levels to the toxic range.
- Management consists of electrolyte correction. Phenytoin is often used for arrhythmias. Antidigitalis antibodies may be used in severe toxicity.

LABORATORY TESTS

Liver Function Tests (LFTs)

- LFTs usually refer to alkaline phosphatase, AST (SGOT), and ALT (SGPT). Some degree of elevation of all three is seen in almost any type of liver pathology. However, severe, or end-stage liver pathology can show low or normal LFTs due to a "burn-out" phenomenon.
- Elevation of the AST and ALT more than the alkaline phosphatase usually indicates liver parenchymal pathology (such as viral hepatitis or alcoholic hepatitis).
- Elevation of alkaline phosphatase out of proportion to the transaminases usually represents an obstructive liver pathology (such as choledocholithiasis). Note that alkaline phosphatase is also produced in other tissues (notably bone), so an isolated increase in alkaline phosphatase may not represent liver pathology at all.
- Alcoholic liver disease usually presents with AST elevation out of proportion to ALT elevation. In addition, the γ-glutamyl transferase (GGT) is also elevated.
- True tests of liver function are more appropriately considered as albumin, PT, PTT, and bilirubin levels. These should be noted in the setting of any increased LFTs.

Renal Function Tests

- BUN and creatinine elevation are seen most commonly in renal disease. Any rise in creatinine should be compared with an old value to determine the chronicity or acuity of the renal impairment.
- A BUN/creatinine ratio of greater than 10 can indicate hypovolemia or dehydration.

- Severely malnourished patients may manifest a decreased BUN level, and this may obscure any usefulness of the BUN/creatinine ratio.
  An acute, isolated rise in BUN may be the first sign of upper GI bleeding.
- Most useful in the work-up of renal failure is the fractional excretion of sodium (Fe_{Na}). A Fe_{Na} less than 1 is usually indicative of prerenal azotemia, whereas a Fe_{Na} greater than 1 points more towards renal etiologies for azotemia. Fe_{Na} is calculated as:

$$\frac{Urinary/Serum\ Na}{Urinary/Serum\ Cr} \times 100$$

Markers of Specific Diseases

- Antinuclear antibody (ANA), is classic for systemic lupus erythematosus, though neither completely specific nor sensitive. Measurement of antibodies to double-stranded DNA (anti-dsDNA) is more specific.
- HLA-B27 is associated with the seronegative spondyloarthropathies, such as ankylosing spondylitis.
- Rheumatoid factor (RF) is associated with rheumatoid arthritis.
- Antimitochondrial antibody is associated with primary biliary cirrhosis.
- Angiotensin converting enzyme (ACE) levels are increased in sarcoidosis.
- Cytoplasmic antineutrophil cytoplasmic antibody (cANCA) is present in Wegener's granulomatosis. Perinuclear antineutrophil cytoplasmic antibody (pANCA) is present in inflammatory bowel disease, primary biliary cirrhosis, and various other disease processes.
- C-peptide is a marker of insulin production, and a low value in the clinical picture of increased insulin state may point to factitious insulin administration.
- Fibrin degradation products (FDP) are elevated in disseminated intravascular coagulation (also look for increased PT/PTT, decreased platelets, and schistocytes on the peripheral blood smear)
- Ham's (acidified serum lysis) test is positive in paroxysmal nocturnal hemoglobinuria.
- Antismooth muscle antibody can be found in chronic active hepatitis, primary biliary cirrhosis, and infectious mononucleosis.

Chapter 5

CARDIOLOGY

Susan L. Taylor, M.D.

CARDIAC MANIFESTATIONS OF SYSTEMIC DISEASES

Coronary Artery Disease (CAD)
- CAD risk factors:
  1. Increasing age
  2. Male sex
  3. Smoking history
  4. Diabetes mellitus
  5. Hypertension
  6. Hypercholesterolemia
  7. Positive family history of CAD

Hypertension
- *CLASSIC PRESENTATION:* Patients with hypertension are usually asymptomatic, however, they may occasionally have headaches or visual changes. Upon physical examination, retinopathy may be found. ECG may reveal left ventricular hypertrophy.
- Hypertension is defined as continuous systolic blood pressure (SBP) greater than 140 mm Hg or diastolic blood pressure (DBP) greater than 90 mm Hg.
- Ninety five % of patients have essential (primary) hypertension. Look for secondary causes in the very young, very old, and those who are refractory to medical therapy.
- Secondary causes of hypertension include oral contraceptive use, renal artery stenosis, intrinsic renal disease, aortic coarctation, primary hyperaldosteronism, Cushing's syndrome, pheochromocytoma, hypercalcemia, alcohol abuse, pregnancy, increased intracranial pressure, and thyrotoxicosis.
- Treat borderline patients with weight loss, decreased alcohol intake, decreased salt in diet, and increased aerobic exercise. Stop oral contraceptives.
- First line drug therapy is usually diuretics, β-blockers, or ACE-inhibitors. Other vasodilators or calcium channel blockers are also used in some cases.

Hypertensive Crisis (Emergency)
- *CLASSIC PRESENTATION:* A patient with a history of hypertension who presents with a SBP greater than 220 mm Hg or a DBP greater than 120 mm Hg. The patient may be asymptomatic or have headaches, seizures, agitation, or a coma. On physical examination there may be retinal changes or papilledema.
- Complications (end organ damage) include hypertensive encephalopathy, intracranial hemorrhage, aortic dissection, myocardial infarction, progressive acute renal failure, or unstable angina.
- If any end organ damage is present, the patient should be admitted to the ICU and treated with parenteral nitroglycerine, nitroprusside, or labetalol.

- Too rapid or too extensive blood pressure reduction can lead to ischemic strokes or blindness.

Hypercholesterolemia

- *CLASSIC PRESENTATION:* An asymptomatic patient is found to have an elevated total cholesterol on routine screening.
- If total cholesterol is less than 200, retest the patient in 5 years.
- If total cholesterol is 200 to 239, the patient has borderline hypercholesterolemia and should be retested in 1 year if the patient has no other coronary artery disease risk factors (see above). If the patient does have other risk factors, a complete lipid profile should be done.
- If total cholesterol is greater than 240, the patient has hypercholesterolemia and a complete lipid profile should be done.
- Persons with borderline hypercholesterolemia should be treated with diet and exercise.
- Drug therapy: HMG-CoA Reductase Inhibitors are usually the drug of choice in initial treatment of hypercholesterolemia. Both HMG-CoA reductase inhibitors and niacin decrease both LDL and triglycerides. Binding resins and probucol primarily decrease LDL, and gemfibrozil primarily decreases triglycerides.

CHEST PAIN AND HEART ATTACK

Angina

- *CLASSIC PRESENTATION:* A middle-aged to elderly patient presents with a "squeezing or tightening" chest pain, beneath or to the left of the midsternum, usually lasting for a few to 15 minutes. The pain increases with physical exertion or stress and subsides gradually with rest or nitroglycerin. The pain may be associated with radiation to the neck or left arm, dyspnea, diaphoresis, or lightheadedness.
- Angina is the symptom of chest pain due to inadequate oxygen supply to the myocardium.
- Angina is classified as:
  Stable – with a predictable and stable pattern of symptoms during exertion that subside with rest. This occurs with a fixed atherosclerotic lesion.
  Unstable – symptoms increase in frequency and/or duration and occur with less exertion and/or even at rest. This generally occurs with a ruptured or thrombosed plaque.
- Treatment for both stable and unstable angina includes smoking cessation, exercise, weight loss, and control of hypercholesterolemia, hypertension, and diabetes mellitus.

- For stable angina, patients should be started on aspirin, a β-blocker, short-acting and/or long-acting nitrates, and in some cases calcium channel blockers.
- For unstable angina, patients should always be admitted. Serial cardiac enzymes and EKGs should be done to rule-out myocardial infarction. The patient should be started on aspirin, heparin, or both (controversial), nitrates IV or transdermal, and β-blockers. Revascularization can be done after the patient's symptoms subside.
- Revascularization can be considered in patients with both stable and unstable angina.
- Coronary artery bypass grafting (CABG) is considered for left main disease or 3-vessel disease with decreasing left ventricular function. There is about a 90% patency rate in 1 year with approximately a 1.5% mortality rate.
- Percutaneous transluminal coronary angioplasty (PTCA) with a balloon catheter used for revascularization has a 30% to 40% incidence of restenosis in 6 months, and is performed in a catheterization laboratory with lower mortality.
- Prinzmetal's (variant) angina is a less common cause of angina that occurs at rest with ST-elevation and a high frequency of associated arrhythmias. This disorder is caused by transient coronary artery spasms. Treat Prinzmetal's angina with nitrates and calcium channel blockers.

Myocardial Infarction (MI)

- *CLASSIC PRESENTATION:* A middle-aged to elderly patient presents with anginal chest pain that is not relieved by rest or nitroglycerin. MI is often accompanied by radiation of the pain to the neck or left arm, diaphoresis, dyspnea, and/or nonspecific anxiety.
- Whereas angina indicates myocardial ischemia (reversible), myocardial infarction causes irreversible damage to the myocardium.
- MIs are frequently silent in diabetics, those on strong analgesics, or those with other neuropathies.
- EKGs of MIs:
    1. Q waves appear in hours to days. With a progressive loss in R waves, these suggest transmural death. The location of the Q waves helps determine the location of the myocardial injury:

        Anterior MI – Q waves in V1-V4. LAD or diagonal branch occlusion with left ventricular dysfunction.
        Inferior MI – Q waves in II, III and AVF. RCA occlusion.
        Posterior MI – Q waves in V1 and V2.
        Lateral MI – Q waves in I, AVL, V5 and V6. LCA occlusion.
    2. ST-segment changes appear in minutes to hours. ST elevation suggests acute injury or active transmural infarction. ST depression suggests ischemia or subendocardial infarction.

3.   T-wave changes appear within minutes to hours. You may see peaked T waves, then T-wave inversion as the MI progresses. T-wave changes are the least reliable indicator of MI.

- Q-wave MIs usually indicate transmural infarction, whereas non-Q-wave MIs are usually subendocardial infarction, although they can be just as dangerous.
- Markers of cardiac damage:
  1.   Creatine phosphokinase (CK) levels are usually elevated in serum after MIs. Detection of the MB isozyme of CK has increased specificity for cardiac muscle, with a high sensitivity.
  2.   Troponin levels are usually increased within 2 hours of an MI, remain elevated longer than CK, and may be a more useful means of diagnosing an acute MI.
  3.   SGOT and LDH levels also rise during the first 24 hours following an MI and decrease over days to weeks.
- Treatment of an acute MI includes:
  1.   Pain relief – Give IV nitrates, then morphine sulfate.
  2.   Clot lysis if within several hours of acute symptoms – streptokinase or tissue plasminogen activator (tPA) are commonly used.
  3.   If thrombolysis is not employed, give heparin, unless it is contraindicated.
  4.   Consider CABG, angioplasty, or intra-aortic balloon pump.
  5.   Daily aspirin, β-blockers.
  6.   Consider calcium channel blockers and/or ACE inhibitors.
  7.   Stool softeners and milk of magnesia, a mild sedative, continuous low-flow oxygen.
  8.   Antihypertensives if appropriate.
  9.   IV diuretics if pulmonary edema is present.
- Complications of an acute MI:
  1.   Ventricular arrhythmias – particularly V-tachycardia and V-fibrillation.
  2.   Cardiogenic shock.
  3.   Supraventricular arrhythmias.
  4.   Heart block.
  5.   Recurrent or persistent ischemia and pain.
  6.   Mechanical complications – left ventricular (LV) rupture, papillary muscle rupture and acute mitral regurgitation, septal rupture, acute tamponade after free wall rupture.
  7.   Emboli – especially with a LV aneurysm.
  8.   Pericarditis.
  9.   Dressler's syndrome occurs in less than 3% of patients. After an acute MI, patients suffer from pericarditis, pleuritis, myalgias, arthralgias, fever, leukocytosis, and an increased sedimentation rate.

Aortic Dissection

- *CLASSIC PRESENTATION:* A patient with a history of hypertension presents with the sudden onset of tearing chest pain that radiates to the back and/or abdomen.
- There may be a murmur of aortic insufficiency on examination.
- Chest x-ray reveals a widened aortic shadow.

Other Causes of Chest Pain

- Pulmonary embolism – See pulmonary section.
- Spontaneous pneumothorax – See pulmonary section.
- Reflux esophagitis classically presents with a burning substernal chest pain of gradual onset. It is usually increased when lying down, and has no change with rest.
- Esophageal spasm classically presents with a squeezing, substernal chest pain, often after meals, and has no change with rest. It is relieved by nitroglycerin.
- Tietze's syndrome (peristernal perichondritis) classically occurs with chest pain that is reproduced by pressure on examination over the sternoclavicular joints. Relieved by aspirin or NSAIDs.
- Hyperventilation syndrome classically presents in an anxious patient, and is usually a sharp chest pain, often with tingling in the fingertips or lips, and lightheadedness. T-wave inversion is common.

Congestive Heart Failure (CHF)

- *CLASSIC PRESENTATION:* An older patient with a history of heart disease presents with fatigue, lethargy, dyspnea on exertion or at rest, paroxysmal nocturnal dyspnea (awakening at night gasping for air), orthopnea (needs extra pillows), weight gain, and/or leg swelling. Physical examination may reveal jugular venous distention, crackles at the lung bases or throughout the lungs, and leg edema.
- CHF occurs when the heart is unable to pump blood in significant amounts at normal filling pressures. CHF may be left-sided (blood backs up to the lungs and pulmonary edema may occur), right-sided (blood backs up to the venous system and leg edema and jugular venous distention may occur), or both.
- Major underlying diseases that can lead to CHF include myocardial infarction, cardiomyopathy, valvular disease, congenital heart disease, hyperthyroidism, and hypertension.
- Acute stressors that can cause CHF exacerbations include acute volume or salt loads, noncompliance with medications, anemia, arrhythmias, infection, hypoxemia, pregnancy, and stress.
- CHF is usually classified based on the cardiac ejection fraction as systolic dysfunction (less than 40% ejection fraction) or diastolic dysfunction (normal ejection fraction, but ventricle is unable to relax for adequate filling during diastole).

- Treatment for early CHF includes salt restriction in the diet, weight loss, and treatment of any exacerbating conditions. Treatment for long-standing CHF includes:
    1. For systolic dysfunction – vasodilators (ACE inhibitors, hydralazine, isosorbide dinitrate) to decrease preload, diuretics, and/or digoxin.
    2. For diastolic dysfunction – diuretics and/or β-blockers to increase ventricular compliance.
- Treatment for acute pulmonary edema is immediate diuretics, nitrates, morphine sulfate, and oxygen. Sit the patient up, and consider albuterol and/or intubation based on circumstances.

Cardiomyopathy

- There are three types of cardiomyopathy, each with different presentations, etiologies, and treatments.

Dilated Cardiomyopathy

- *CLASSIC PRESENTATION:* A patient in CHF with a dilated ventricle, or with arrhythmias.
- Etiologies include infection (viral – Coxsackie B, echovirus; parasitic – Chagas' disease), idiopathic, chronic coronary artery disease, alcohol, toxins (doxorubicin), postpartum, and infiltrative diseases.
- Treat with warfarin to prevent emboli, diuretics, and by decreasing afterload (ACE-inhibitors, nitrates, or hydralazine).

Restrictive Cardiomyopathy

- *CLASSIC PRESENTATION:* A patient in CHF with pulmonary or systemic venous congestion, along with increased diastolic pressures.
- Etiologies include amyloidosis and endomyocardial fibrosis.
- There is no effective therapy, but calcium channel blockers may increase diastolic compliance.

Hypertrophic Cardiomyopathy

- *CLASSIC PRESENTATION:* A patient with angina, exertional syncope, dyspnea, and/or sudden death.
- The patient has restricted ventricular filling and outflow obstruction.
- Valsalva maneuvers will increase the obstruction and any murmur.
- Etiology is usually familial, with autosomal dominant inheritance. Treat with β-blockers or calcium channel blockers.

PERICARDITIS AND ATRIAL FIBRILLATION

Etiologies of Pericarditis

*   Infection
    1.   Viral infection is most common. This is usually benign and self-limited.
    2.   Bacterial infection is less common. Purulent bacterial infection has a 50% mortality. Tuberculosis can also cause pericarditis.
*   Uremia
*   Blunt chest trauma
*   Myocardial infarction
*   Connective tissue diseases (e.g., systemic lupus erythematosus)
*   Neoplasms – especially lung, breast, lymphoma and malignant melanoma

Acute Pericarditis

*   *CLASSIC PRESENTATION:* A patient presents with sharp and stabbing pain in the chest or across the top of the shoulders. The intensity of the pain is affected by respiration and position. On physical examination there is a friction rub, best heard during expiration and with the patient leaning forward.
*   EKG may show ST elevation and T-wave inversion.
*   Important note: A person with slow, gradual, chronic pericarditis may have up to a few hundred milliliters of fluid in their pericardium and be asymptomatic. A person with acute onset pericarditis will usually become symptomatic with less than 50 milliliters of fluid in the pericardium, because they have not had time to compensate.
*   Treat suspected viral pericarditis with bedrest and analgesia. The patient may respond to corticosteroids.

Pericardial Tamponade

*   *CLASSIC PRESENTATION:* A patient with the same symptoms as acute pericarditis, and tachycardia. Later this patient is noted to have a drop in blood pressure, with quiet or muffled heart sounds. Patients may sometimes also have *pulsus paradoxus* (a decrease in systolic blood pressure of greater than 10 with inspiration).
*   Patients have increased venous pressures and decreased arterial pressures. Ventricular filling is decreased, usually with a pericardial effusion. Cardiac output is decreased.
*   Treat by increasing cardiac output with large volume infusions IV followed by pericardiocentesis.

Constrictive (Chronic) Pericarditis

- *CLASSIC PRESENTATION*: Patients do not frequently present with chest pain. Usually they present with signs of increased venous pressure such as ascites and peripheral edema, as well as fatigue. They do not usually have pulmonary edema. They may have atrial fibrillation.
- Kussmaul's sign (an inspiratory rise in jugular venous pressure) may be seen on physical examination.
- Chest x-ray usually reveals a small heart and lungs, sometimes with calcifications around the heart. Chronic inflammation causes scars, calcifications, and adherence of the pericardium to the myocardium.
- Treat by surgically stripping the pericardium.

Atrial Fibrillation

- *CLASSIC PRESENTATION*: An older patient who presents with fatigue, dyspnea, palpitations, chest pain, dizziness, and/or syncope. Alternatively, some patients present with few or no symptoms. Upon examination the patient is found to have an irregularly irregular pulse. An EKG reveals no P-waves and an irregularly irregular ventricular response.
- Etiologies of atrial fibrillation include:
    1. Cardiac causes – sick sinus syndrome, Wolff-Parkinson-White syndrome (WPW), coronary artery disease, congestive heart failure, cardiomyopathy, myocarditis, congenital heart disease, hypertension (just about any cardiac disease).
    2. Pulmonary causes – pulmonary embolism.
    3. Pericardial disease.
    4. Hyperthyroidism.
    5. Intoxication – alcohol, β-agonists, theophylline.
    6. Infection.
    7. Postoperative.
    8. Idiopathic.
- The main complication is a 5% per year risk of stroke. The risk of stroke is further increased with CHF, hypertension, a dilated right atrium, and a previous history of stroke.
- Treatment of atrial fibrillation includes:
    1. Rate control
        a. cardioversion - indicated with rapid a-fib and life-threatening problems, contraindicated if the patient is not yet anticoagulated or an atrial thrombus is not ruled out by transesophageal echocardiography.

       b.   AV node blockers – digoxin, diltiazem, verapamil, esmolol. Contraindicated in WPW syndrome or any other wide-complex tachycardia.

       c.   Chronic rate control medications – β-blocker or digoxin.

2. Chronic rhythm control – procainamide, quinidine, amiodarone.
3. Anticoagulation to prevent stroke – warfarin or aspirin (for low-risk patients).

Chapter 6

SURGERY

Sergio Huerta, M.D.

TRAUMA

Resuscitation

- The main goal of a trauma team in resuscitation is to keep the brain alive in the face of vital organ failure.
- Brain survival depends on adequate oxygenation, so the aim of resuscitation is to maintain adequate brain perfusion. In the Advanced Trauma Life Support (ATLS) protocol, the steps in resuscitation are as follows.
    1. Revival
    2. Examination of vital functions
    3. Definitive care

Revival

- The required order of steps involved in revival can be remembered easily by the following mnemonic.

    A = airway
    B = breathing
    C = circulation
    D = decompression
    E = exposure
    F = fluids

Airway

- Management of the airway involves ensuring that there is a clear path for air to get into the lungs.
- Assessment should include presence of an obstruction (e.g., dentures or blood) in the airway.
- In the unconscious patient, the most common obstruction is the patient's own tongue, which can be quickly cleared by chin lift and/or jaw thrust.
- If the patient is conscious, spoken words demonstrate airway patency.
- Care should be taken with the patient suspected of having neck injury when establishing airway patency so as not to exacerbate neurological damage. In this case, the jaw should not be elevated and spinal immobilization should be performed.

Breathing

- Once a clear airway has been established, appropriate breathing should be assessed.
- Inspection of the chest as it rises should indicate air movement. This may be followed by auscultation of the lungs for inflow/outflow of air.
- If the patient is not moving air, ventilation should be started.

- Flail chest usually occurs when there are multiple rib fractures resulting in paradoxical movement of the chest with respiration. Intubation with positive pressure ventilation should be promptly started.
- Cardiac tamponade occurs when there is bleeding into the pericardial cavity resulting in impaired cardiac contractions. The diagnosis is a clinical one and consists of decreased heart sounds, increased jugular venous pressure (JVP), and decreased blood pressure (Beck's triad). With cardiac tamponade, immediate IV fluids and pericardiocentesis should be performed.

Circulation
- Circulation is quickly assessed by carotid or femoral pulse palpation.
- Presence of either of these pulses ensures a systolic blood pressure of at least 60 mm Hg even in the absence of radial pulses.
- Capillary refill (< 2 seconds) and skin color are also good indicators of adequate perfusion.
- If pulses are not palpable, cardiopulmonary resuscitation (CPR) should be started.
- Once airway, breathing and circulation have been adequately attended, a brief history should be obtained form the patient or relatives. The mnemonic AMPLE can be used to remember required information for a quick history from the trauma patient.

    A = allergies
    M = medications
    P = past medical history
    L = last meal
    E = events preceding the emergency

Decompression
- The trauma patient should receive gastric decompression with an NG tube. This reduces the risk of aspiration in patients with emesis.
- Decompression of the bladder should also be done by placement of a Foley catheter. A Foley catheter is a reliable way to assess urine output and thus adequate hydration status.

Exposure
- Complete disrobing of the patient allows a complete examination by inspection and palpation of the trauma patient.

Fluids
- Aggressive fluid resuscitation should be done in the trauma patient to keep urine output greater than 50 ml/hr.

- For most situations, Ringer's lactate or normal saline are adequate fluids to resuscitate the trauma patient. These can be given as rapid infusions until urine output is within the normal range.
- If urine output remains low even after 4 liters of fluid, or if the patient remains hypotensive, blood products should be considered in the resuscitative effort.

After Revival
- Following revival, the trauma patient should be closely examined from head to toe.
- Vital functions and a brief neurological examination should also be performed.
- The Glasgow coma scale is useful in determining neurological injury, but need not be memorized for the purposes of USMLE, Step 2.
- The next step includes appropriate studies such as radiographic films, diagnostic peritoneal lavage to determine the presence of abdominal lesions, and CT scan as necessary.

COMMON TRAUMA COMPLICATIONS

Hypovolemic Shock
- Hypovolemic shock occurs as a result of vascular contraction due to decreased blood volume. This may be as a result of bleeding or severe dehydration. However, in the trauma patient, hypovolemic shock should be assumed to be due to bleeding.
- Dry mucous membranes, decreased jugular venous pressure, and tachycardia are common manifestations of hypovolemic shock.
- Treatment should be aimed at volume repletion. There should be a low threshold to give O⁻ blood products in this scenario.

Cardiogenic Shock
- Cardiogenic shock occurs as a result of failure of the heart to pump (i.e., CHF).
- In contrast to hypovolemic shock, patients in cardiogenic shock have evidence of fluid overload (i.e., elevated JVP and edema).
- Fluid should be administered with extreme caution in these patients.
- Treatment may include afterload reduction with diuretics, as well as cardiotonic drugs such as dobutamine.

Neurogenic Shock
- Neurogenic shock occurs due to loss of vascular tone following spinal cord injury.
- Treatment is aimed at increasing the peripheral vascular resistance with vasoconstrictive drugs.

Septic Shock
- Septic shock occurs as a result of endotoxin release by bacteria.
- Broad-spectrum antibiotics should be quickly administered to treat the infectious process.

Pneumothorax
- *CLASSIC PRESENTATION:* A trauma patient with tachypnea, pleuritic chest pain, and hypotension. An x-ray will show decreased pulmonary vasculature where the lung has deflated.
- A chest tube should be inserted to relieve the pressure on the lung and allow re-expansion of the lung.

Cardiac Tamponade
- *CLASSIC PRESENTATION:* A patient with decreased heart sounds, elevated JVP, and decreased blood pressure.
- Immediate pericardiocentesis should be performed to remove the fluid from the pericardial cavity.

BENIGN BREAST DISEASE

General
- The female breast is composed of glandular, ductal, connective, and fatty tissue.
- Fibroglandular tissue refers to the composite of dense fibrous stroma and functional lobules and ducts.
- The 12 to 14 lobules are responsible for the production of milk, which is carried to the nipple by the array of ducts. These structures are supported by the stroma composed of connective tissue, Cooper's ligaments, and fat.
- In the reproductive years the amount of fibroglandular tissue predominates over fat. Fibroglandular tissue responds to estrogen and progesterone, which are responsible for the cyclic changes in the postmenstrual phase.
- After menopause, this tissue begins to involute and is replaced by fat, which makes mammography more sensitive.
- The major lymphatic drainage of the breast is to the axilla. Minor drainage occurs to the parasternal nodes, which run with the internal mammary artery.
- Supraclavicular and contralateral nodes are not within the normal path of lymphatic drainage. Thus, involvement of these nodes with a tumor indicates poor prognosis.

Disorders of the Breast

- For the table below, the distribution of breast disorders in women complaining of a breast mass are shown. Thus, of the women complaining of breast mass, 40% will have fibrocystic changes.

DISORDERS OF THE BREAST	PERCENTAGE
Fibrocystic Changes	40%
No disease	30%
Benign tumors	13%
Cancer	10%
Fibroadenoma	7%

Fibrocystic Condition

- *CLASSIC PRESENTATION:* A female patient with a complaint of breast tenderness and "lumpiness" that follows a cyclical monthly pattern.
- Fibrocystic condition is a descriptive term that encompasses the following changes in the breast.
    1. Cyst formation
    2. Glandular or connective tissue hyperplasia
    3. Lymphatic infiltration
    4. Stromal fibrosis
    5. Apocrine metaplasia or hyperplasia
    6. Sclerosing adenosis
- Fibrocystic changes are the most common lesions affecting the female breast, most often in the 30- to 50-year-old group.
- One of the hallmarks of this condition is its cyclic nature, often associated with monthly breast tenderness.
- The breast tenderness may be due to the physiological response of fibroglandular tissue to menstrual hormonal changes as breast engorgement and tenderness occur within 1 week before and after the menstrual period.
- Most fibrocystic changes do not have an associated risk for cancer.
- The management of fibrocystic changes is conservative and consists of regular follow-up and symptomatic treatment for tenderness.
- Decreasing caffeine intake, reduction of tobacco use, and ingestion of vitamin E have also been advocated to ameliorate breast tenderness.

- If there is a mass associated with fibrocystic changes, ultrasound can usually discriminate between its cystic or solid nature. If uncertainty still exists, fine-needle aspiration (FNA) is indicated.
- Cysts usually disappear following FNA. Solid masses require further work-up if their nature is uncertain.

Fibroadenomas

- *CLASSIC PRESENTATION:* A young female who presents with a well-defined, smooth, firm, mobile breast mass that is nonpainful.
- Fibroadenomas are encapsulated fibromas that are easily recognized on physical examination by their specific character consisting of a well-defined, smooth, firm, mobile masses.
- They usually occur in the 20- to 30-year-old female group.
- Fibroadenomas also respond to hormonal stimulation and may grow during pregnancy.
- There is no risk of malignancy with fibroadenomas. These can be followed conservatively.
- However, surgical excision is an option because fibroadenomas can grow and some may harbor a sarcoma such as cystosarcoma phyllodes.

BREAST CANCER

General

- One in 10 women will develop breast cancer.
- Risk factors for carcinoma of the breast include age, radiation exposure, history of breast or breast-ovarian cancer in first-degree relatives (mother, sister, daughter).
- About 5% of all women with breast cancer may have a germ-line mutation(s) in the BRCA1 gene.
- Carriers of the BRCA1 gene may have an 85% lifetime risk of breast cancer with 50% of the breast cancers occurring prior to age 50 years.
- Early menarche, nulliparity, or late child-bearing also appears to be minor risk factors.

Clinical Presentation

Symptoms	Signs
Breast mass (most common presentation)	Mass (palpable range > 1 cm)
Asymptomatic	Edema
Nipple retraction and discharge	Lymphadenopathy: axillary (the most common metastasis) supraclavicular (indicates poor prognosis)
Edema (due to lymphatic blockage)	

Evaluation
- The evaluation of breast disease begins with a through history and physical examination (H&P).
- The table above indicates some salient elements that should be obtained with the H&P.
- Important aspects in the history may include being over the age of 40, a family history of breast or ovarian cancer in first-degree relatives, a previously abnormal mammogram, a previous history of breast cancer, and any change in a breast mass.
- Aspects of the physical examination that suggest breast cancer include breast asymmetry, edema, discoloration, skin changes, ulceration, nipple discharge, and nipple retraction. Axillary or supraclavicular lymphadenopathy are also suggestive of cancer.

Diagnosis
- Any breast mass requires a prompt diagnosis because treatment options and management are highly dependent on the type and stage of the cancer.
- Definitive diagnosis is made by tissue biopsy and histopathology.
- Several modalities may be used to evaluate a breast mass.

Mammography
- Mammograms are radiological images of the breast that are used for screening purposes in the asymptomatic patient from age 40 to 50 years.
- In the symptomatic patient, mammograms only increase or decrease the suspicion of cancer.
- Mammography can also be used to guide the surgeon to obtain a biopsy in nonpalpable masses.

- Other forms of screening include breast self-examination (BSE) and physical examination by a physician.
- The American Cancer Society recommendations for breast cancer screening are as follows.

Age	Screening and frequency
>20	Breast self-examination every month
20 to 40	Physical examination every 3 years
>40	Physical examination every year
40 to 50	Mammogram every other year
>50	Mammogram every year

Ultrasonography
- Ultrasound is a noninvasive test that can quickly discriminate between solid and cystic masses.

Fine-Needle Aspiration (FNA)
- Aspirated cells are evaluated to determine if malignancy is present.
- FNA can also determine the presence or absence of estrogen receptors (ER) and progesterone receptors (PR). Normal breast tissue contains high quantities of ER and PR that allow it to respond to menstrual hormones.
- Absence of receptors indicates poor prognosis because hormone chemotherapy (tamoxifen) is not possible.
- One of the limitations of FNA is that it can not assess tumor invasion. Thus, further tests are required.

Excisional Biopsy
- Excisional biopsy provides assessment of the margins, invasiveness, and receptor status.

Core-needle Biopsy
- Core-needle biopsy involves the removal of several cores of tissue to evaluate tissue architecture, which provides information about tumor invasion.

Common Sites of Metastasis
- Lymph nodes (75%)
- Lungs (70%)

- Bone (60%)
- Liver (60%)
- Brain (15%)

Types of Breast Cancer

- About 90% of breast cancers arise from the ductal system.
- The remaining 10% arise from the lobules. Thus, breast cancers are either named ductal or lobular.
- Some important types of cancers are discussed below.

Infiltrating (Invasive) Ductal Carcinoma

- Infiltrating ductal carcinoma is the most common type of malignancy of the female breast.
- Because of its hard consistency due to the increased fibrous tissue stroma, this type of cancer is also called scirrhous carcinoma. The connective tissue is responsible for dimpling of the skin and retraction of the nipple.
- See below for treatment options.

Lobular Carcinoma *in Situ* (LCIS)

- LCIS is a noninvasive cancer.
- Women with LCIS have a nine-fold higher risk of developing breast cancer than the general female population.
- These lesions are usually picked up as incidental findings because there are most often no signs and symptoms. Treatment consists of close follow-up.

Ductal Carcinoma *in Situ* (DCIS)

- DCIS is also known as intraductal carcinoma without invasion.
- These tumors usually do not cause distant metastasis, but can infiltrate the ductal system and produce extensive lesions.
- DCIS cancers are thought to be precursors for invasive cancer.
- Treatment may consist of removal of tumor with clear margins, lumpectomy with or without radiation, or mastectomy, depending on the size of the tumor.

Paget's Disease

- Paget's disease of the nipple is a form of ductal carcinoma.
- Treatment consists of mastectomy or removal of nipple and areolar complex with negative margins.

Inflammatory Carcinoma

- Inflammatory carcinoma is a very aggressive form of breast cancer characterized by rapid enlargement of the breast, with erythema, warmth, and pain.

- This type of cancer requires aggressive multimodality treatment (see below).

Treatment Options for Breast Cancer

- Surgery is the form of treatment of most cancers at an early stage.
- Chemotherapy, hormonal therapy, and radiotherapy along with surgery is recommended for more advanced disease.
- The role of surgery in advanced disease is primarily palliation. Surgical options for early disease include the following.
    1. Radical mastectomy, which involves removal of all breast, pectoralis muscles, and axillary contents. There is a high morbidity associated with radical mastectomy and it is seldom used anymore.
    2. Modified radical mastectomy involves removal of all breast and axillary contents without pectoralis muscles. This is the most commonly applied treatment and has the same survival benefit as radical mastectomy.
    3. Breast conservation therapy, which includes segmental mastectomy, quadrantectomy, or lumpectomy, differs primarily by the amount of breast tissue removed.
    4. This technique also includes removal of the breast tumor with negative margins, axillary dissection, and breast irradiation.
    5. Contraindications to breast conservation therapy include: patients whose cancers cannot be excised with negative margins, patients who cannot receive radiation therapy, multicentric tumors, and a tumor that is large relative to breast size.

- Advanced cancers may require the following therapies.
    1. Chemotherapy is indicated for all breast cancers that have nodal involvement.
    2. Hormonal manipulation is used when the tumor is positive for ER or PR. Therapies include tamoxifen in postmenopausal women. Premenopausal women may undergo bilateral oophorectomy to remove the endogenous source of estrogen.
    3. Radiation therapy may be effective for treating local disease.

THE ACUTE ABDOMEN

General

- An acute abdomen is the acute onset of abdominal pain in an otherwise healthy individual.
- A previously healthy individual who develops abdominal pain that persists for more than six hours should be evaluated by a surgeon to determine if the patient

needs to go to the operating room. The decision regarding the need for immediate, urgent, or elective surgery is a major challenge.

- The following are conditions that should be excluded rapidly in a patient who develops acute abdominal pain as they require immediate surgical intervention.
    1. Ruptured aneurysm
    2. Ruptured ectopic pregnancy
    3. Spontaneous splenic or hepatic rupture
    4. Hemodynamic instability
- The following conditions should also be excluded because they require urgent surgical intervention.
    1. Appendicitis (most common cause of acute abdomen)
    2. Perforated viscus
    3. Strangulated hernia
    4. Mesenteric necrosis
    5. Peritoneal signs
- The following diagnoses should be entertained because they may require elective surgical intervention.
    1. Cholecystitis
    2. Diverticulitis
- The following criteria are used to establish the severity of the abdominal pain and the need for surgical intervention.
    1. History of pain
        a. onset (acute vs. gradual)
        b. character (sharp vs. dull)
        c. duration
        d. frequency
        e. location
        f. aggravation of alleviating factors and associated symptoms
    2. Physical examination (see below)

Common Signs of an Acute Abdomen

- Murphy's sign is associated with an inflamed gallbladder. There is a positive Murphy's sign when pain and an arrest of inspiration is elicited with palpation of the right upper quadrant.
- The obturator sign is associated with appendicitis. The patient with a positive obturator sign experiences suprapubic pain with internal rotation of the hip.
- The psoas sign is associated with appendicitis. A positive psoas sign occurs when there is suprapubic pain with extension of the hip.
- Rovsing's sign is also associated with appendicitis. This occurs when rebound palpation of the left lower quadrant produces pain in the right lower quadrant
- Costovertebral angle tenderness is associated with kidney pathology (e.g., stones or pyelonephritis).

Differential Diagnosis of Abdominal Pain by Quadrant

Right Upper Quadrant	Left Upper Quadrant
1. Stomach 　　PUD 　　Perforated ulcer 　　Gastritis 2. Gallbladder 　　Cholelithiasis 　　Choledocholithiasis 　　Cholecystitis 　　Cholangitis 3. Pancreas 　　Pancreatitis 4. Liver 　　Hepatic abscess 　　Liver tumors 　　Hepatitis 5. Lungs 　　Lower lobe pneumonia	1. Stomach 　　PUD 　　Perforated ulcer 　　Gastritis 　　Reflux 2. Spleen 　　Rupture 　　Abscess 3. Thoracic 　　Pneumonia 　　PE 　　Dissecting aortic aneurysm 4. Kidney 　　Pyelonephritis 　　Nephrolithiasis 5. Hiatal Hernia 6. Trauma 　　Boerhaave's syndrome 　　Mallory-Weiss tear

Right Lower Quadrant	Left Lower Quadrant
1. Small bowel and appendix 　　SBO 　　Meckel's diverticulum 　　Appendicitis 　　Intussusception 2. Pancreatitis 3. Colon 　　Diverticulitis 　　Volvulus 　　Perforated viscus 　　Colon CA 　　Inflammatory bowel disease 4. Renal 　　UTI 　　Nephrolithiasis 5. Ruptured AAA 6. Gynecologic 　　Ectopic pregnancy	1. Small bowel and appendix 　　SBO 　　Appendicitis 　　Intussusception 2. Colon 　　Diverticulitis 　　Volvulus 　　Perforated viscus 　　Colon CA 　　IBD 3. Renal 　　UTI 　　Nephrolithiasis 4. Ruptured AAA 5. Gynecologic 　　Ectopic pregnancy 　　PID 　　Mittelschmerz 　　Ovarian torsion/tumor

Upper Gastrointestinal (GI) Bleeding

- *CLASSIC PRESENTATION:* A patient who presents with hematemesis, melena (black, tarry stool), hematochezia (bright red blood per rectum in massive upper GI bleeding), Guaiac-positive stool, epigastric discomfort, weakness, or syncope. Any of the above symptoms may be present.
- GI bleeding is classically classified as an upper GI bleeding if it occurs above the ligament of Treitz (located at the junction of duodenum and jejunum) and lower GI bleeding for bleeding distal to the ligament of Treitz.
- After ensuring hemodynamic stability and patient stability, it is important to establish if the source of bleeding is from the upper or lower GI tract.
- NG tube suction can include or exclude upper GI bleeding.
- If NG tube aspiration is positive for blood, upper GI endoscopy should be the next step in identifying the source of bleeding.
- Upper GI endoscopy is especially useful in identifying esophageal varices and peptic ulcer disease.
- If NG tube aspiration is negative for blood, anoscopy/proctoscopy should be performed.
- ^{99m}Tc-labeled red blood cells and selective angiography can also be used to detect the source of bleeding.
- Common causes of upper GI bleeding

1.	Duodenal ulcer	(25%)
2.	Gastric ulcer	(20%)
3.	Acute gastritis	(15%)
4.	Mallory-Weiss tear	(10%)
5.	Esophageal/gastric varices	(8%)

- Treatment includes fluid resuscitation, NG suction, water lavage, and surgery as needed.

Lower Gastrointestinal Bleeding

- *CLASSIC PRESENTATION:* Symptoms may be similar to those for upper GI bleeding and include melena, hematochezia, pallor, diaphoresis, and confusion. In cases of acute loss, there may be tachycardia, postural hypotension, systolic hypotension, and syncope. Bright red blood per rectum is more common in lower GI bleeding. Melena is more common in upper GI bleeding because blood mixes with stool along the GI tract.
- Common causes of lower GI bleeding

  1. Diverticulosis
  2. Vascular ectasia
  3. Colon cancer
  4. Polyps
  5. Ischemic/infectious colitis
  6. Inflammatory bowel disease

7. Hemorrhoids

- If lower GI bleeding is suspected, anoscopy and rigid sigmoidoscopy should be performed.
- Use of ^{99m}Tc-labeled RBC is the test of choice to identify the source of lower GI bleeding.
- Vasopressin is usually used as a temporary measure to resuscitate the patient before proceeding with further management.
- Embolization may also stop acute bleeding but should be reserved for patients who are poor surgical candidates because it carries a 15% complication rate.
- If a patient requires more than two thirds of their circulating blood volume in less than 24 hours or if there is hemodynamic instability, laparotomy is indicated to identify and stop the source of bleeding.

THE ESOPHAGUS

Type I (Sliding) Hiatal Hernia
- *CLASSIC PRESENTATION:* A patient who presents with symptoms of gastroesophageal reflux disease (GERD), including burning epigastric pain and substernal tightness. The symptoms are exacerbated by gastric irritants such as alcohol, tobacco, and caffeine. Many patients note a sensation of food being stuck in the esophagus.
- Type I hiatal hernia occurs when the distal esophagus and proximal stomach herniate through the esophageal hiatus in the diaphragm.
- Type I hiatal hernia is 100 times more common than Type II.
- Although patients present with GERD, these are separate disorders.
- Risk factors for the development of hiatal hernias are associated with increased abdominal pressure, such as obesity and pregnancy.
- Diagnosis is established by esophageal manometric testing, which measures pressures on both sides of the diaphragm and will demonstrate a loss of the high-pressure area at the lower esophageal sphincter.
- Barium swallow, esophageal pH testing, and endoscopy may also be helpful.
- Two thirds of patients respond to medical therapy, which includes avoidance of gastric irritants, weight loss, avoidance of food intake for several hours before going to bed, sleeping with the head elevated 30 degrees, and regular use of antacids.
- Surgical therapy is aimed at correcting the anatomic defect and preventing reflux by increasing the pressure at the lower esophagus.

Type II (Paraesophageal) Hiatal Hernia
- *CLASSIC PRESENTATION:* Type II hernias usually are asymptomatic unless they incarcerate and become ischemic. In this case, the patient will experience dysphagia and bleeding.

- In Type II hernias, the esophagogastric junction is in the correct position; however, a portion of the gastric fundus herniates through a defect in the diaphragm next to the esophagus.
- Reflux is uncommon with paraesophageal hernias.
- On chest x-ray, air-fluid levels may be seen in the posterior mediastinum.
- Barium swallow helps identify anatomic abnormalities.
- Surgery is indicated for patients with Type II hernias since incarceration and strangulation may occur. Thirty percent of untreated hernias lead to catastrophic events.
- Surgery consists of reduction of the hernia and repair of the hiatal defect.

Reflux Esophagitis
- *CLASSIC PRESENTATION:* A patient with symptoms of GERD, including burning, nonradiating epigastric pain and substernal tightness, which are exacerbated by gastric irritants such as tobacco, alcohol, and caffeine (essentially the same symptoms as Type I hiatal hernia).
- The pathogenesis of reflux esophagitis is unclear, but it is thought to be multifactorial. Possible causes include weakness of the lower esophageal sphincter, short intra-abdominal esophageal length, and increased abdominal pressure due to obesity or pregnancy.
- The disease in caused by long-standing exposure of the esophagus to gastric acid rather than the amount of acid present.
- Complications include mucosal erosion, ulceration, stricture, and aspiration pneumonia.
- Chronic gastroesophageal reflux may result in Barrett esophagus, which occurs when the epithelium of the distal esophagus undergoes metaplasia from the normal stratified squamous epithelium to columnar epithelium more typical of the stomach.
- The risk of developing adenocarcinoma in patients with Barrett esophagus is 50 to 100 times higher than the normal population.
- Treatment of Barrett esophagus consists of treatment of reflux, which does not reverse the metaplasia but prevents its progression.
- The management of reflux esophagitis is primarily medical, which is essentially the same as that for Type I hiatal hernia.
- If medical management fails, surgery is indicated to increase the pressure around the lower esophageal sphincter.

Achalasia
- *CLASSIC PRESENTATION:* A patient who presents with dysphagia, regurgitation of undigested food, and weight loss. There may be a history of aspiration pneumonia.

- Achalasia is the most common motility disorder of the esophagus. It occurs when the lower esophageal sphincter (LES) fails to relax during swallowing.
- Achalasia may lead to the formation of scattered esophageal diverticula.
- Contrast studies reveal dilation of the proximal esophagus and diverticula.
- Manometry shows diffuse spasm of the esophagus with hypertonic activity at the LES.
- Treatment includes surgical transection (myotomy) or balloon dilatation of the LES.
- Treatment of diverticula consists of excision and treatment of the underlying disease.

Zenker's Diverticula

- *CLASSIC PRESENTATION:* A patient with the complaint of chronic halitosis and the regurgitation of recently swallowed food, accompanied by choking.
- Zenker's diverticula are outpouchings in the cervical esophagus, secondary to esophageal motility disorders such as achalasia.
- The treatment is excision of the diverticula and myotomy of the cricopharyngeal muscle.

Esophageal Cancer

- *CLASSIC PRESENTATION:* A patient with a history of smoking, drinking, or achalasia who presents with dysphagia, pain, and weight loss. Contrast radiography may show the typical "apple core" lesion in the esophagus.
- Squamous cell carcinoma is the most common esophageal malignancy, followed by adenocarcinoma.
- Risk factors for squamous cell carcinoma include tobacco and alcohol use, achalasia or diverticula of the esophagus, and poor oral hygiene. Squamous cell carcinoma is more common in African Americans.
- Risk factors for adenocarcinoma include Caucasian heritage, gastroesophageal reflux, and Barrett esophagus.
- The symptoms of esophageal cancer are usually insidious and generally occur after the disease has progressed significantly leading to poor prognosis.
- Diagnosis is made by barium swallow and endoscopy with biopsy.
- Surgical resection is the mainstay of treatment for the lower one third of the esophagus.
- Radiotherapy is the primary form of treatment for cancers arising in the upper esophagus.
- Chemotherapy may improve the 5-year survival rate but the overall cure rate for esophageal cancer is only about 5%.

Boerhaave's Syndrome

- *CLASSIC PRESENTATION:* A patient with a history of recent vomiting who presents with dysphagia, chest or abdominal pain, diaphoresis, tachycardia, and respiratory distress.
- Boerhaave's syndrome is a form of esophageal perforation that occurs following emesis and involves all layers of the esophagus.
- The syndrome occurs frequently in alcoholics following emesis against a closed epiglottis.
- The diagnosis is made by chest x-ray or esophagram with water-soluble contrast medium.
- Treatment includes broad spectrum antibiotics and surgical repair of the esophageal perforation.

Mallory-Weiss Syndrome

- *CLASSIC PRESENTATION:* A patient with epigastric or thoracic substernal pain and hematemesis following retching or vomiting (note the lack of systemic symptoms that are seen in Boerhaave's syndrome).
- The diagnosis is made by history, physical, and endoscopy. X-ray may reveal a pneumothorax.
- Treat with water lavage to stop bleeding. Electrocautery or arterial embolization may be necessary to stop the bleeding.

DISORDERS OF THE STOMACH

Peptic Ulcer Disease (PUD)

- *CLASSIC PRESENTATION:* A 40- to 60-year-old patient who presents with a complaint of epigastric pain that is exacerbated by fasting and improved by taking antacids or food.
- PUD occurs when the protective mechanisms of the gastrointestinal tract are unable to deal with acid secretion, which leads to mucosal erosion.
- Peptic ulcer disease refers to both gastric and duodenal ulcers, which have different characteristics.
- *Helicobacter pylori* has been identified in 90% of patients with duodenal ulcer disease and about 70% of patients with gastric ulcer disease.
- Tobacco smoking is a big risk factor for the development of PUD, and smoking cessation often helps the problem.

Duodenal Ulcers

- Duodenal ulcers occur as a result of excessive acid secretion. Duodenal ulcers occur two times more often than gastric ulcers and occur more commonly in men.

- The clinical presentation of duodenal ulcers depends on the severity and duration of the ulcers as well as presence of complications. The following complications are observed in duodenal ulcers.
    1. Hemorrhage
    2. Obstruction
    3. Perforation
- Massive bleeding may occur if the ulcer erodes into the gastroduodenal artery. The signs of massive bleeding are primarily hemodynamic (decreased blood pressure, increased heart rate, and syncope).
- Perforation may also produce the signs and symptoms of an acute abdomen.
- In the presence of perforation, an x-ray typically reveals the presence of free air.
- *H. pylori* infection may be detected with the urea breath test or by antibody detection.
- An upper gastrointestinal series, which consists of barium swallows, may be done.
- Endoscopy is even more accurate than an upper gastrointestinal series and may be therapeutic as well.
- Gastric acid analysis consists of nasogastric tube placement in the stomach and acid collection every 15 minutes for 2 hours. Patients with PUD usually have high basal acid output.
- The medical treatment for duodenal ulcers consists of the following.
    1. *H. pylori* eradication with any of a number of antibiotic regimens. A common one is bismuth subsalicylate, metronidazole, and tetracycline for 2 weeks.
    2. Smoking cessation.
    3. Decrease the intake of irritants such as caffeine, chocolate, and alcohol.
    4. Antacids.
    5. Anticholinergic agents.
    6. H_2-blockers such as cimetidine and famotidine.
    7. H^+ pump inhibitors such as omeprazole.
- Surgical treatment is indicated if a duodenal ulcer is complicated by intractability, obstruction, hemorrhage, or perforation.
- Patients suspected of perforation or a patient requiring more than six units of blood in 24 hours should undergo exploratory laparotomy.
- If upper GI bleeding is suspected, decompression of the stomach with an NG tube should follow. Treatment includes ligation or embolization of the affected vessel.

Gastric Ulcers
- *CLASSIC PRESENTATION:* A middle-aged patient who presents with epigastric pain that is exacerbated by the ingestion of food (in contrast to duodenal ulcers, which are ameliorated by food).
- Weight loss may be a part of the clinical presentation.

- Gastric ulcers have an unclear etiology, though *H. pylori* infection is a frequent component.
- Other possible mechanisms include a defective mucus barrier and delayed gastric emptying.
- The hydrochloric acid load is normal to mildly elevated.
- Gastric ulcers usually occur in the lesser curvature of the stomach.
- In contrast to duodenal ulcers, gastric ulcers may be associated with malignancy.
- Diagnosis may be made with an upper GI series or endoscopy. However, because of the associated risk of malignancy with gastric ulcer, multiple biopsies should be taken during endoscopy.
- Compared to duodenal ulcers, a smaller percentage of gastric ulcers respond to medical treatment.
- The medical treatment is similar to that for duodenal ulcers, except anticholinergic drug therapy is contraindicated in gastric ulcers because slowing gastric emptying time is counter-productive.
- Prostaglandin-blocking medications such as aspirin or steroids should be discontinued.
- Surgical therapy such as distal gastrectomy with excision of the ulcer is generally successful in the majority of the cases with a very small recurrence rate.

Zollinger-Ellison Syndrome

- *CLASSIC PRESENTATION:* A patient who has had a problem with recurrent intractable duodenal ulcers.
- This syndrome is caused by the direct production of gastrin by a tumor usually arising in the pancreas or paraduodenal area. About two thirds of these tumors are malignant.
- The diagnosis is made by gastrin serum levels above 300 pg/ml.
- Medical management consists of H_2-blockers and proton pump inhibitors.
- Surgery may be performed if an isolated identifiable tumor is localized. If the tumor is not localized, proximal gastric vagotomy in combination with medical treatment is indicated.
- Definitive treatment consists of total gastrectomy as this entirely eliminates the source of acid.

Gastric Cancer

- *CLASSIC PRESENTATION:* A patient with a history of epigastric pain, weight loss, dysphagia, hematemesis, and melena.
- The incidence of gastric cancer in the United States is low compared to Japan, China, and Finland.
- Environmental and dietary factors have been advocated as possible etiologic agents.
- The majority of gastric carcinomas originate in the distal half of the stomach.

- Risk factors for the development of gastric cancer include gastric polyps, chronic gastritis, pernicious anemia, and gastric ulcer disease.
- Metastatic disease occurs to regional lymph nodes, omentum, and the left supraclavicular area (Virchow's node).
- Diagnosis is made by upper GI series or endoscopy with biopsy.
- The surgical treatment is complete surgical resection of the stomach and regional resection as necessary.
- The 5-year survival rate depends on the stage of the cancer. The 5-year survival rate in the United States is about 10%, due to the late diagnosis of gastric carcinoma.

THE SMALL INTESTINE

Small Bowel Obstruction (SBO)

- *CLASSIC PRESENTATION*: A patient who presents with intermittent crampy abdominal pain, nausea and vomiting, constipation, and abdominal distension. High-pitched bowel sounds are classically heard on physical exam.
- The patient may also have obstipation, which is the inability to pass flatus. This occurs in cases of complete bowel obstruction.
- There are often fluid and electrolyte imbalances, most commonly hypokalemic metabolic alkalosis, secondary to fluid loss into the intestinal lumen.
- If perforation of the bowel has occurred, the patient may present with signs and symptoms of peritonitis and sepsis.
- There may be a history of previous surgeries or cancer. The physical examination should investigate the presence of hernias.
- Small bowel obstruction may be differentiated from paralytic ileus and large bowel obstruction by using the table below.
- An acute abdominal series (AAS) (upright chest, supine abdomen-KUB, and upright abdomen films) is the most useful study to establish the diagnosis.
- Barium enema is also used in the diagnosis of SBO if there is still uncertainty with the AAS studies.
- Patients with complete bowel obstruction should undergo exploratory laparotomy because a major risk with SBO is the development of strangulation.
- The goals of surgical intervention are to relieve the obstruction and to resect any necrotic small intestine.

	Small Bowel Obstruction	Paralytic Ileus	Large Bowel Obstruction
Common Causes	Adhesions (60%) Hernia (20%) Tumor (15%) Intussusception Crohn's disease (5%)	Acute pancreatitis Appendicitis Cholecystitis Gastroenteritis	Colon cancer Diverticulitis Volvulus
History and Physical Examination	Crampy abdominal pain Nausea and vomiting Constipation and obstipation High-pitched bowel sounds or absent in complete obstruction	Minimal continuous abdominal pain Nausea and vomiting Constipation and obstipation Absent bowel sounds	Crampy abdominal pain Nausea and vomiting Constipation and obstipation High-pitched or absent bowel sounds
AAS Findings	Dilated loops of small bowel occupying center of abdomen Small, closely spaced mucosal folds Little or no colonic gas Differential air-fluid levels	In prone position, air will flow to rectum if no obstruction. Thus there are large amounts of gas in the small intestine and colon.	Dilated loops of bowel occupying periphery of abdomen Widely spaced haustra

Adenocarcinoma of the Small Bowel

- *CLASSIC PRESENTATION:* Adenocarcinoma typically causes intermittent or partial small bowel obstruction.
- Adenocarcinoma is the most common malignancy of the small bowel, yet represents only 1% of all GI cancers.
- The diagnosis of adenocarcinoma is made by the finding of occult blood in the stool and by barium studies or endoscopy.
- The treatment is wide surgical excision of the tumor and mesenteric lymph nodes.
- Due to the typically late diagnosis, the 5-year survival rate is only 20 to 30%.

Carcinoid Tumors

- *CLASSIC PRESENTATION:* A patient who presents with cutaneous flushing, bronchospasm and wheezing, chronic watery diarrhea, and valvular heart disease (the carcinoid syndrome).
- Carcinoid tumors produce large amounts of serotonin, which account for many of the symptoms.
- Carcinoid tumors are cancers of neuroectodermal origin; thus, they are also known as APUDomas (**A**mine **P**recursor **U**ptake and **D**ecarboxylation).
- They have high potential for metastasis and are malignant.

- The small bowel is the second most common location for these tumors. More than 50% of carcinoid tumors occur in the appendix.
- Clinically significant findings include elevated serum serotonin levels and urine 5-HIAA levels.
- Medical therapy includes octreotide infusion and chemotherapy.
- Surgical therapy is excision of the tumor, though this has not been shown to affect survival rates.

Lymphoma

- *CLASSIC PRESENTATION:* A patient with anorexia and weight loss, anemia, and small bowel obstruction (nonspecific findings).
- Lymphoma represents the most common malignancy of the small bowel in the pediatric population.
- Lymphoma commonly occurs in the ileum.
- Treatment is wide surgical excision including mesenteric lymph nodes and chemotherapy.

BILIARY TRACT DISEASE

Common Lesions of the Biliary Tract

- Cholelithiasis is the formation of gallstones in the gallbladder.
- Cholecystitis is inflammation of the gallbladder. It is caused most commonly by obstruction of the cystic duct by gallstones, leading to bile stasis, inflammation, and possibly infection.
- Acalculus cholecystitis occurs in about 10% of the cases of cholecystitis. It usually occurs in the hospitalized patient in whom stimuli to secrete bile has been impaired by prolonged fasting, TPN, trauma, or severe dehydration resulting in bile stasis and inflammation.
- Empyema of the gallbladder is a complication of cholecystitis that results in a pus-filled gallbladder.
- Choledocholithiasis is the complete or partial obstruction of the common bile duct by gallstones.
- Cholangitis is a bacterial infection of the biliary tract due to obstruction.
- Suppurative cholangitis is a severe infection of the biliary tract with "pus under pressure."

Cholelithiasis and Cholecystitis

- *CLASSIC PRESENTATION:* An overweight, middle-aged female patient who presents with intermittent right upper quadrant pain after eating, which radiates to the scapula. This symptom may be accompanied by nausea and vomiting.
- Jaundice may be present if there is obstruction of the common bile duct.

- The intermittent right upper quadrant pain is referred to as biliary colic.
- Murphy's sign is caused by an inflamed gallbladder and is an arrest of inspiration with palpation of the right upper quadrant.
- Charcot's triad (in cases of cholangitis) is jaundice, fever, and chills.
- Reynold's pentad (in cases of acute suppurative cholangitis) is Charcot's triad with altered mental status and hypotension.
- Eighty percent of biliary calculi are asymptomatic.
- Risk factors for the development of cholesterol stones are the classic four Fs: Female, Fertile, Forty, Fat.
- Seventy-five percent of gallstones are made of cholesterol and 25% are made of bile pigments.
- The risk factors for bile pigment stones are hemolytic disorders, cirrhosis, and bile stasis.
- Complications of cholelithiasis include cholecystitis, choledocholithiasis, cholangitis, gallstone pancreatitis, gallstone ileus, gallbladder necrosis, and biliary fistulas.
- Common laboratory findings include an elevated white blood count, increased direct bilirubin, increased alkaline phosphatase, and increased AST/ALT.
- Diagnosis is made by ultrasonography which detects gallstones in 95% of the cases.
- Percutaneous transhepatic cholangiography (PTC) involves injection of contrast media directly into the intrahepatic duct and is the most sensitive test for delineating biliary anatomy and obstruction.
- Endoscopic retrograde cholangiopancreatography (ERCP) is diagnostic and therapeutic for biliary obstruction.
- Cholelithiasis is treated by elective cholecystectomy and is recommended for symptomatic cholelithiasis in the absence of complications.
- Patients with a calcified gallbladder have a 50% risk of developing carcinoma of the gallbladder and should have it removed.
- Cholecystectomy can be performed by open or laparoscopic surgery. The latter has less morbidity and mortality than the former.
- Cholecystitis is treated with antibiotics, NG decompression, and cholecystectomy.

DISEASES OF THE PANCREAS

Acute Pancreatitis
- *CLASSIC PRESENTATION:* A patient with constant epigastric pain radiating to the back, accompanied by nausea and vomiting. Physical examination reveals fever, tachycardia, right upper and lower quadrant tenderness, absent bowel sounds, and rebound tenderness. There is an elevated serum amylase and lipase.

- Laboratory values indicative of acute pancreatitis are leukocytosis, elevated amylase levels (a sensitive test), and elevated lipase levels (a specific test).
- Acute pancreatitis occurs when there is an acute inflammation of the pancreas caused by release and activation of pancreatic enzymes causing parenchymal destruction.
- Most of the causes of acute pancreatitis can be remembered by the mnemonic BAD SHIT.

    B = Biliary calculi

    A = Alcoholism

    D = Drugs (furosemide, steroids, thiazides, estrogens)

    S = Scorpion bites (one of the least common causes of acute pancreatitis)

    H = Hyperparathyroidism (hypercalcemia) and hyperlipoproteinemias

    I = Infections (mumps, Coxsackie virus, Epstein-Barr virus, rubella, hepatitis A and B)

    T = Trauma (blunt and penetrating trauma, ERCP)

- Biliary calculi and alcoholism account for 85% of acute pancreatitis. Ten percent are idiopathic.
- Complications of acute pancreatitis include necrotizing pancreatitis (15% of cases), pancreatic abscess (2% of cases), paralytic ileus, and pseudocyst formation.
- The diagnosis of acute pancreatitis is facilitated by a history (especially with a history of alcohol abuse or gallstones) and physical examination. Elevated amylase and lipase levels are almost pathognomonic.
- Abdominal films may show a paralytic ileus, pancreatic calcifications, or the presence of gallstones (in 10% of cases).
- Ultrasound may reveal inflammation, gallstones, a pseudocyst, or pancreatic abscess.
- Medical management includes making the patient NPO, fluid resuscitation, and pain relief.
- Surgical intervention may be required for exploratory laparotomy to remove gallstones and drain pancreatic abscesses.

Chronic Pancreatitis
- *CLASSIC PRESENTATION:* A patient with steatorrhea and intermittent epigastric pain after food.
- Chronic pancreatitis occurs when there is permanent destruction of pancreatic parenchyma resulting in fibrosis, calcification, and loss of endocrine and exocrine function.
- The loss exocrine function results in steatorrhea.
- The loss of endocrine function results in the signs and symptoms of diabetes mellitus.

- Common causes of chronic pancreatitis include alcoholism, hyperparathyroidism hyperlipidemia, cystic fibrosis, and trauma.
- Diagnosis may be facilitated by elevated amylase/lipase levels, stool fat analysis, and glucose levels (serum/urine).
- CT scan demonstrates glandular enlargement/atrophy, ductal enlargement, calcification, masses, pseudocysts, inflammation, or extension beyond the pancreas.
- Medical treatment includes alcohol cessation, treatment of hyperparathyroidism if indicated, insulin to treat diabetes mellitus, and pancreatic enzyme replacement.
- Surgical therapy is often pancreatojejunostomy.

Pancreatic Carcinoma

- *CLASSIC PRESENTATION:* The presentation depends on the location of the tumor within the pancreas. (See table below)

Head of the pancreas	Body or tail
Painless jaundice Palpable nontender gallbladder (Courvoisier's sign Pruritus Dark urine Increased direct bilirubin Increased alkaline phosphatase	Nausea and vomiting Weight loss and fatigue Migratory thrombophlebitis Jaundice

- Pancreatic cancer is the fifth most common cancer in the United States, with a 2:1 male predominance.
- The greatest risk factors for pancreatic cancer are age and cigarette smoking.
- The most common type (90%) is poorly differentiated adenocarcinoma from the ductal epithelium.
- Two thirds of pancreatic cancers arise from the head of the pancreas.
- There is a very poor survival rate (5 to 10% 5-year survival rate despite surgical intervention).
- There is frequently an elevated bilirubin/alkaline phosphatase due to biliary obstruction.
- The diagnosis is made by CT scan, ultrasound, or ERCP with biopsy.
- If the tumor is in the body or tail of the pancreas, the treatment is distal resection of the pancreas.
- If the tumor is in the head of the pancreas, a Whipple procedure is performed.

LOWER GI TRACT: COLON AND RECTUM

Diverticular Disease
- Diverticula are pouches off the lumen of a tubular organ. They occur in all segments of the GI tract, but occur most commonly in the colon.
- True diverticula are outpouchings in the bowel wall involving all of its layers. True diverticula are not common and are usually congenital.
- False diverticula are outpouchings of the bowel wall involving only the mucosal and submucosal layers. False diverticula are the most common type in the colon and more than 90% occur in the sigmoid colon.
- Diverticulosis is one or more diverticula in the colon.
- Diverticulitis is inflamed diverticulosis.

Diverticulosis
- *CLASSIC PRESENTATION:* Most patients with uncomplicated diverticulosis are asymptomatic. A patient may present with bright red blood per rectum (BRBPR) or, on occasion, left lower quadrant abdominal pain and a change in bowel habits.
- Lower GI bleeding with a change in bowel habits is more suggestive of colon cancer.
- Patients presenting with bright red blood per rectum are at risk of massive bleeding if the bleeding is due to diverticulosis.
- Complications of diverticulosis include diverticulitis (20%) and diverticular bleeding (5 to 10%).
- When diverticulosis is complicated by diverticulitis or diverticular bleeding, a workup consisting of barium enema and colonoscopy (this should be done at least 6 weeks after the acute phase of the clinical complication) should be performed.
- The management of uncomplicated diverticulosis is conservative and consists of a high-fiber diet.
- The management of diverticular bleeding is outlined in the lower GI bleeding section.

Diverticulitis
- *CLASSIC PRESENTATION:* An older patient who presents with left lower quadrant abdominal pain, constipation or diarrhea, fever, and leukocytosis.
- Complications of diverticulitis include perforations, abscess formation, bowel obstruction, and fistula formation.
- The diagnosis is made primarily by history and physical examination. Barium enema and colonoscopy should not be performed during the acute phase of the disease due to risk of perforation.
- An acute abdominal series (AAS) may reveal signs of free air (suggesting perforation) or dilated loops and air-fluid levels (suggesting obstruction).

- The initial management of diverticulitis without complications includes bowel rest and IV antibiotics with Gram-negative coverage.
- Recurrent episodes of diverticulitis may require elective sigmoidectomy.
- Diverticulitis presenting with an acute abdomen (perforation, abscess, or obstruction) may require exploratory laparotomy if the patient is hemodynamically unstable. Surgical resection of the affected colon may be required. An older patient with diverticulitis should be followed closely. A younger patient should undergo sigmoidectomy because the probability of recurrence is high.

Colonic Polyps
- *CLASSIC PRESENTATION:* Polyps that have not evolved into carcinoma are usually asymptomatic. However, some polyps may present with bleeding or a change in bowel habits such as diarrhea or constipation.
- A polyp is a mucosal and/or submucosal growth into the lumen of the bowel.
- Premalignant polyps are adenomas.
- Polyps can be sessile (flat and closely attached to the mucosal surface) or pedunculated (round and attached to the mucosal surface by a thin neck).
- The presence of polyps is usually established while screening for other conditions such as colon cancer or inflammatory bowel disease (IBD) by barium enema or colonoscopy.
- Once the presence of polyps has been established, removal by colonoscopy is indicated. Histologic evaluation should be performed to exclude the possibility of cancer.
- If a polyp is found to be adenomatous, a full colonoscopy should be performed to exclude the presence of any other polyps in the rest of the colon.

Familial Adenomatous Polyposis (FAP)
- FAP is an autosomal dominant disease with nearly complete penetrance in which affected individuals develop hundreds of adenomatous polyps in the colon and rectum beginning early in adolescence, inevitably progressing to colon cancer if untreated.
- FAP occurs as a result of a mutation of the adenomatous polyposis coli (APC) gene.
- Patients with family history of FAP should be followed closely for the development of polyps. Those with polyps should undergo prophylactic colectomy.

Gardner's Syndrome
- Gardner's syndrome is a variant of FAP in which there are extraintestinal manifestations such as desmoid tumors, osteomas of the skull, and sebaceous cysts in addition to the usual hundreds of adenoumatous colonic and rectal polyps.
- Gardner's syndrome is also an autosomal dominant disease, but it has variable penetrance.

Turcot's Syndrome

- Turcot's syndrome is a variant of FAP consisting of colonic polyps and CNS gliomas or malignant melanoma.

Peutz-Jeghers Syndrome

- *CLASSIC PRESENTATION:* A patient who presents with mucocutaneous pigmentation and is found to have hamartomatous polyps throughout the GI tract.
- Extraintestinal malignancy of the ovaries, breast, and thyroid are also associated with this syndrome.

Colon Cancer

- *CLASSIC PRESENTATION:* An older patient who presents with rectal bleeding, weight loss, bowel obstruction, or a change in bowel habits. Abdominal pain may or may not be present. A CBC reveals that the patient is anemic.
- A change in stool caliber is suggestive of left-sided colon cancer.
- Obstruction is uncommon with right-sided colon cancer.
- Colorectal carcinoma is the fourth most common cancer and the second leading cause of death in the United States.
- Most deaths occur because colorectal cancer is usually diagnosed by symptomatology, when the disease has advanced to an aggressive stage.

The distribution of colon cancer is shown in **Figure 6.1**.

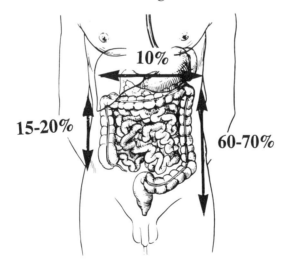

10%

15-20%

60-70%

Figure 6.1

- Risk factors for colon cancer include the following.
    1. Ulcerative colitis (the risk is 5 to 10% at 20 years and 15 to 20% at 30 years).
    2. First-degree relatives with colon cancer.
    3. Familial adenomatous polyposis (FAP). Nearly all patients with FAP will develop colon cancer before the age of 40 if untreated.

4.   The incidence increases significantly by age 50 and peaks at age 70.
5.   High-fat/low-fiber diet.

- The work-up for colon cancer begins with a good history and a digital rectal examination with hemoccult testing for the presence of blood in the stool.

- The next step is flexible sigmoidoscopy/colonoscopy or barium enema.

- In patients in whom colon cancer has been detected, preoperative full colonoscopy is indicated to detect synchronous lesions.

- Carcinoembryonic antigen (CEA) is an adhesion molecule that is over-expressed in the great majority of colon cancers. This is not a screening test but should be obtained preoperatively to determine the baseline level and assess recurrence after surgery.

- Liver function tests (LFTs) should be obtained as part of the preoperative laboratory tests in order to assess possible metastasis to the liver.

- The mainstay for the treatment of colon cancer is surgical resection. Surgical resection includes removal of the involved segment with at least a 5 cm margin, its lymph nodes, and its blood supply.

- 5-fluorouracil (5-FU) and levamisole lower morality by about 30% in patients with Dukes stage C disease.

- Colon cancer recurrence is high. Therefore, follow-up should include the following.
   1.   Physical examinations every 1 to 2 months
   2.   CEA level determination every 2 months after surgery
   3.   Colonoscopy or barium enema every 6 months after surgery for the first 2 years

Inflammatory Bowel Disease (IBD)

- Ulcerative colitis and Crohn's disease constitute the inflammatory bowel diseases.
- The etiology of these disorders in not understood.
- There is an increased incidence in Jewish populations and a decreased incidence in African-American populations.
- Complications of IBD include fistula formation and colonic perforation (more common with Crohn's disease), as well as hemorrhage, obstruction, toxic megacolon, and colon cancer (more common with ulcerative colitis).
- The medical treatment of both ulcerative colitis and Crohn's disease is with sulfasalazine and steroids.
- Sulfasalazine is taken up by affected tissue and then converted to aminosalicylate, which is anti-inflammatory.
- Steroids have many side effects, should only be used during an acute flare-up and should be gradually discontinued soon after resolution of the acute flare-up.
- Surgical intervention is indicated when medical treatment fails or complications occur. Surgery is usually palliative.

- Surgical intervention in ulcerative colitis is usually performed due to intractability of the disease in which case surgery is therapeutic.
- Differences exist in both of these disorders, which are important in helping to make a diagnosis.

Characteristic	Ulcerative Colitis	Crohn's Disease
GI distribution	Limited to the colon (colitis) and rectum (may lead to megacolon)	Involves the entire GI tract from anus to mouth Colon > small bowel
Course	More frequent flare-ups with periods of remission	Indolent and chronic
Pattern along GI tract	Continuous	Intermittent with skipped lesions
Bowel wall involvement	Limited to the mucosa	Entire wall
Response to medical therapy	Fairly good	Fairly poor
Colon cancer risk	High	Low

Ulcerative Colitis
- *CLASSIC PRESENTATION:* A patient who presents with bloody diarrhea, weight loss, fever, abdominal pain.
- The bloody diarrhea is due to the mucosal involvement of the lesion.
- Ulcerative colitis has more flare-ups with periods of remission.

Crohn's Disease
- *CLASSIC PRESENTATION:* A patient who presents with weight loss, fever, diarrhea, and symptoms of intestinal perforation or fistula formation.
- Perianal fistulas are especially common.
- Diagnosis is made by colonoscopy or barium enema.

Hemorrhoids
- *CLASSIC PRESENTATION:* (internal hemorrhoids are above dentate line): A patient who presents with the complaint of rectal discomfort, bleeding, and prolapsing tissue.
- *CLASSIC PRESENTATION:* (external hemorrhoids are below dentate line): A patient who presents with severe rectal pain and prolapsing tissue.
- The severe pain in external hemorrhoids is due to thrombosis of the hemorrhoid.

- Internal hemorrhoids are further classified into four different types.
    1. First degree hemorrhoids are those that do not prolapse.
    2. Second degree hemorrhoids prolapse but spontaneously reduce.
    3. Third degree hemorrhoids require manual reduction
    4. Fourth degree hemorrhoids cannot be reduced.
- Risk factors associated with the development of symptomatic hemorrhoids are constipation, excessive exercise, and pregnancy.
- Low-fiber diet may also play a role in the development of hemorrhoids.
- Diagnosis is made by inspection of the rectal and perineal area, and examination with an anoscope as needed.
- The medical management of hemorrhoids includes stool softeners, stool bulking agents, sitz baths, and topical anesthetics.
- Surgical treatment of bleeding internal hemorrhoids (third and fourth degree) includes rubber band ligation or surgical resection.

THE APPENDIX

Acute Appendicitis

- *CLASSIC PRESENTATION:* A patient who presents with pain that began in the periumbilical region and localized to the right lower quadrant of the abdomen, with nausea and vomiting that followed the onset of the pain. Anorexia is a very important component.
- Low-grade fever, positive psoas (pain on extension of right hip), obturator (pain on rotation of the hip), and Rovsing's signs (pain in RLQ during rebound palpation of LLQ), and leukocytosis (10,000 to 20,000 cells/μl) are other indicators of acute appendicitis.
- The right lower quadrant tenderness classically occurs one third of the distance from the anterior superior iliac spine to the umbilicus (McBurney's point).
- Appendicitis occurs due to inflammation of the appendix caused by narrowing of its lumen.
- Narrowing may be caused by hyperplasia of the appendix (commonly seen in children) or by fecal material (fecalith), which is commonly seen in young adults.
- Acute appendicitis is the most common cause of acute abdomen.
- Two of the following three elements must be present for a diagnosis of acute appendicitis.
    1. Right lower quadrant abdominal pain (must be present along with one of the other two following)
    2. Appropriate history (including anorexia)
    3. Leukocytosis (10,000 to 20,000 cells/μl)
- If the diagnosis is still uncertain, an acute abdominal series may help rule out other diagnoses. In 5% of the cases a fecalith can be observed in plain films. Plain

films are also useful in assessing the possibility of perforation by looking for free air in the abdomen.
- Ultrasound or CT may also be helpful in making a diagnosis.
- Untreated appendicitis may lead to perforation in less than 24 hours. Therefore, clinical suspicion of acute appendicitis requires prompt surgical intervention.
- Preoperative antibiotics to cover aerobic (and anaerobic if perforation is suspected) bacteria may be administered.
- Postoperative antibiotics for the first 24 hours if perforation has not occurred and for 7 days in the case of perforation.

Cancer of the Appendix
- The most common type of cancer of the appendix is carcinoid tumor.
- These malignant cancers originate from APUD cells (neural crest derivatives) and are also known as APUDomas.
- These tumors secrete large amounts of serotonin producing cutaneous flushing, bronchospasm and wheezing, valvular heart disease (and right-sided heart failure), and chronic watery diarrhea (carcinoid syndrome).
- Often, cancer of the appendix is an incidental finding during appendectomy.
- Laboratory findings include elevated serum serotonin and elevated 5-HIAA in the urine.
- An appendectomy is usually performed if the tumor is less than 2 cm and a right hemicolectomy is performed if the carcinoid tumor is larger than 2 cm.
- Medical therapy includes octreotide (somatostatin agonist) infusion.

Meckel's Diverticulum
- *CLASSIC PRESENTATION*: Meckel's diverticulum has a variety of presentations which include intestinal hemorrhage (especially in children), intestinal obstruction, inflammation, and incarcerated/strangulated hernias.
- Meckel's diverticulum is a remnant of the embryonic vitelline duct. This is the most common congenital anomaly of the small bowel.
- The diagnosis is made primarily by history and physical examination.
- An acute abdominal series may rule out other causes of abdominal pain or bleeding.
- Barium and radionuclide studies may be required if there is suspicion of bleeding.
- Symptomatic Meckel's diverticulum should be resected.
- Meckel's diverticulum is often described as a "disease of twos".
    1. Occurs in about 2% of adults
    2. Symptomatic in about 2% of patients
    3. Symptoms usually present before 2 years of age
    4. Occurs about 2 feet from the ileocecal valve
    5. About 2 inches long
    6. M:F ratio is 2:1

7.   Contains 2 types of ectopic tissue (gastric and/or pancreatic)
8.   Has 2 major complications (hemorrhage and inflammation)

ABDOMINAL HERNIA

General

- *CLASSIC PRESENTATION:* A patient with a mobile mass that appears, sometimes intermittently, in the groin. There is occasional discomfort and pain associated with the mass. In males, there may be a mass in the scrotum, and this is best palpated by maneuvers that increase intra-abdominal pressure.
- It may be possible to reproduce the symptoms of a hernia by voluntarily increasing abdominal pressure, e.g., with a Valsalva maneuver or coughing in a standing position.
- In some hernias the only presenting symptoms may be those of bowel obstruction.
- An abdominal hernia is the protrusion of all or part of a structure through a defect in the abdominal wall. It can be congenital, acquired or iatrogenic.
- Irreducible hernias warrant urgent attention because they may incarcerate.

Indirect Inguinal Hernia

- An indirect inguinal hernia (most common type in men and women, more often on the right) passes through the internal ring of the inguinal canal and travels toward the external ring.
- It may enter the scrotum upon exiting the external ring.
- Patency of the processus vaginalis is required but not sufficient for its formation.
- The risk of strangulation is higher with indirect hernias than with direct hernias.

Direct Inguinal Hernia

- This is a hernia that protrudes through the *trigonum inguinale* (Hasselbach's triangle), formed by the deep epigastric artery, the inguinal ligament, and the rectus sheath.
- It contains no peritoneal sac.
- It is an acquired type of hernia.

Femoral Hernia

- Femoral hernias protrude through the femoral ring, which is limited medially by the lacunar ligament, posteriorly by Cooper's ligament, and anteriorly by the inguinal ligament.
- This is an acquired lesion.
- Femoral hernias contain no peritoneal sac.
- This is the type of hernia most susceptible to incarceration and strangulation.

Hernia type	Male	Female	Children
Direct	40%	Rare	Rare
Indirect	50%	70%	100%
Femoral	10%	30%	Rare

Other Types of Abdominal Hernia

- An incisional hernia is a hernia through an incisional site. It usually occurs as a result of incomplete closure of previous abdominal surgery and subsequent development of an infection at this site.

- Richter's hernia is an incarcerated or strangulated hernia involving only one side of the bowel wall. Because the lumen of the bowel is still patent, bowel necrosis may occur in the absence of bowel obstruction.

- An obturator hernia occurs as a protrusion of abdominal structures through the obturator canal. These are much more common in females.

NECK MASSES

General

- Neck masses are either congenital, inflammatory, or neoplastic.
- The clinical manifestations of a neck mass depend on type as shown in the table below.

	Congenital	Inflammatory	Neoplastic
Age of onset	birth-young adult	child-young adult	adult
Type of onset	persistently present	recent, short duration	chronic onset, slow growth
Characteristic of mass	soft, painless	soft	firm, solid
Symptoms	stridor, dyspnea, dysphagia	fever, pain/tenderness, erythema	weight loss, stridor, dyspnea, dysphagia, +/- pain
Predisposing factors	none	varied	alcohol, tobacco

Congenital Neck Masses

- The following are common congenital masses.
    1. Thyroglossal duct cyst
    2. Dermoid cyst
    3. Pharyngeal cleft cyst
    4. Cystic hygroma
    5. Hemangioma
- These masses are characteristically soft, painless, persistent, and seen early.
- Thyroglossal duct cysts and dermoid cysts occur in the midline.
- Pharyngeal cleft cysts occur laterally in the neck.
- Cystic hygromas are multilocular masses that compress underlying structures.
- Hemangiomas may be located in the oral cavity, parotid gland, or neck, and characteristically enlarge with crying.
- All are treated with surgical excision, except hemangioma, which typically regresses by age 5.

Inflammatory Masses

- Inflammatory masses are the most common type of neck masses affecting children and young adults.
- Symptoms of infection such as fever, pain/tenderness, and erythema are common characteristics of these masses.
- Common inflammatory masses are the result of an infectious agent typically in the salivary glands or lymph nodes and include viral lymphadenitis, bacterial adenitis, Ludwig's angina (a bacterial infection that results from dental infections), and fungal adenitis occurring in the immunocompromised patient.
- Viral infections are generally self-limited.
- Bacterial infections require appropriate antibiotics, and surgical debridement on occasion.
- Fungal infections require amphotericin B and surgical debridement.

Neoplastic Masses

- *CLASSIC PRESENTATION*: A patient with a history of heavy alcohol or tobacco use who presents with a progressively enlarging, firm, solid neck mass. This type of neck mass should be considered neoplastic unless proved otherwise.
- Neoplastic masses can be benign or malignant.
- The most common benign masses occurring in the neck include lipomas and neurogenic tumors.
- Lymphoma is the most common malignant neoplasm in children and young adults.
- In adults with a history of alcohol and tobacco use, the most common type of malignancy is squamous cell carcinoma.
- Benign masses require surgical excision.
- Malignant neoplasms require radiation, surgery, or both.

- Most midline tumors in both children and adults are in the thyroid gland. Benign thyroid masses include Graves' disease and toxic thyroiditis. Malignancies of the thyroid may arise from follicular cells, C-cells, or lymphoid tissue (lymphoma).
- Papillary carcinoma is the most common type of thyroid CA.
- Medullary carcinoma (arising from C-cells) is often genetically transmitted and it is associated with the multiple endocrine neoplasm syndrome (MEN syndrome). This cancer carries a poor prognosis.
- Surgery is the treatment of choice for thyroid cancer.
- Treatment with iodine 131 (^{131}I) may be used for those cancers that concentrate iodine (papillary and follicular carcinoma).

MEN Syndromes

MEN I	MEN IIa	MEN IIb
• Parathyroid hyperplasia • Pituitary adenoma • Pancreatic tumors	• Medullary carcinoma • Pheochromocytoma • Parathyroid hyperplasia	• Medullary carcinoma • Pheochromocytoma • Mucosal neuromas • Marfanoid habitus

Diagnosing Neck Masses
- Ultrasound is useful in establishing the cystic or solid nature of a neck mass.
- CT is indicated if the nature of the mass is uncertain.
- Fine-needle aspiration (FNA) can, in most cases, establish a definitive diagnosis of a neck mass.
- Biopsy is indicated in patients where a diagnosis is not possible by other means.

ORTHOPEDIC SURGERY

Definitions
- A bone fracture is a break anywhere in a bone.
- A subluxation is the partial loss of contact of joint surfaces.
- A dislocation is the complete loss of contact of joint surfaces.

Common Fractures
- Closed fractures are fractures in which the skin remains intact.

- Open fractures are fractures in which there is communication of the bone with the external environment. This includes pelvic fractures that may communicate with the rectum or vagina and are not readily visible by rapid inspection. These are contaminated and mandate aggressive treatment.
- A greenstick fracture is a fracture that is incomplete. Only one side of the bone (one cortex) is disrupted. This occurs most commonly in children.
- A stress fracture is a fracture caused by repeated stress on a bone.
- A pathologic fracture is a fracture that occurs in a diseased bone (e.g., in osteoporosis).
- A simple fracture generates only two bone fragments.
- A comminuted fracture generates more than two bone fragments.
- Fractures involving the epiphyseal plate have the potential to cause growth disturbances.

Clinical Manifestations and Management

- Symptoms of fracture include pain, swelling, and deformity.
- Fractures involving nearby blood vessels may present with decreased or absent pulses and hemodynamic manifestations.
- Fractures with nerve injury may present with sensory or motor deficits.
- Diagnosis is usually made with a history, physical examination, and x-ray in two views.
- The patient should be assessed for vascular and/or nervous involvement.
- All fractures should be splinted as soon as possible after assessment of ABCs.
- Reduction involves the restoration of bone alignment.
- Closed reduction is the alignment of the bones by manipulation without surgical exposure of the bones.
- Open reduction is the alignment of the bones with surgical exposure of the bone fragments. An open fracture should be managed by the open reduction method.
- The reduction may be maintained by casting, traction, internal fixation, or external fixation.
- All open fractures are contaminated by definition and require immediate intervention, including IV antibiotics, tetanus prophylaxis, and surgical debridement. This should be followed by open reduction and internal fixation.
- Other indications for open reduction of fractures include intra-articular fractures, closed reduction failure, and vascular or neural involvement.

Orthopedic Emergencies

- Orthopedic emergencies include the following.
    1. Open fractures
    2. Compartment syndrome
    3. Fractures with vascular/neural involvement
    4. Bone/articular infections (osteomyelitis/septic arthritis)

5.   Hip fractures

Compartment Syndrome

- *CLASSIC PRESENTATION:* A patient with recent injury to a limb who presents with the 4 **P**'s: **P**ain, **P**aresthesia, **P**allor, and **P**aralysis of the limb.
- Pulses may be present even in severe cases of compartment syndrome and should not be used to rule out compartment syndrome.
- Compartment syndrome is the drastic increase in pressure of muscle groups, which are normally enclosed in osseo-fascial compartments.
- Common causes of compartment syndrome include fractures, muscle contusions, and crush injuries.
- Compartment pressure may be so elevated that muscle necrosis may ensue.
- The diagnosis of compartment syndrome is made if compartment systolic pressure is greater than 30 mm Hg, though a high degree of suspicion is sufficient to initiate treatment.
- Compartment syndrome is treated by immediate decompression by open fasciotomy.

NEPHROLITHIASIS

Overview

- *CLASSIC PRESENTATION:* A male patient with the acute onset of severe flank pain radiating to the groin, often accompanied by nausea and vomiting. The patient may not be able to sit still. Patients may also present with urinary frequency, urgency, and hematuria.
- Urinary calculi (stones) may be caused by urine supersaturation with calcium oxalate or uric acid and subsequent crystallization. If the crystals are trapped, they quickly form stones.
- Formation of stones leads to obstruction. Common sites of obstruction are the uretopelvic junction, uretovesicular junction, and the intersection of the ureter and the iliac vessels.
- Renal calculi affect one in 100 people (more often males).

Types of Stones

- Calcium oxalate stones comprise 75% of all stones and are radiopaque. They are often associated with an increased dietary calcium or a history of hyperparathyroidism.
- Struvite stones comprise 15% of all stones. They are associated with urinary tract infections and are described as "staghorns." The urine will have a pH > 7.2.
- Uric acid stones comprise 7% of all stones and cannot be seen on x-ray. They are often associated with a history of gout.

- Cystine stones comprise 1% of all stones.

Evaluation

- The history should provide information about diet, history of hyperparathyroidism, or family history of nephrolithiasis.
- On physical examination, there will be severe flank tenderness.
- Urinalysis and urinary culture reveal hematuria, WBCs, RBCs.
- CBC reveals ↑ WBC and ↑ BUN/creatinine ratio.
- Kidney-ureters-bladder (KUB) plain films often reveal visible stones. Eighty percent of calculi can be detected by plain films of the abdomen.
- Serum calcium and parathyroid hormone may be elevated.

Radiodensities

Calcium oxalate	Struvite	Cystine	Uric acid

⟶

Radiopaque			Radiolucent

Diagnosis

- The diagnosis is made by KUB or intravenous pyelogram (IVP) -- contrast material is injected IV, which collects in the urinary system and an x-ray of the abdomen is taken.

Management

- Hemodynamic stability should be assessed because patients may be volume depleted following nausea and vomiting. Appropriate hydration should be rapidly started.
- Pain control should be initiated with morphine or meperidine.
- Treatment of urinary stones is largely dependent on the type, size, and location of the stone.
- Calcium Oxalate stones greater than 5 mm may case obstruction. These stones do not respond well to hydration or alkalization of the urine.
  1. If the stone is located in the kidney, extracorporeal shock-wave lithotripsy (ESWL) often causes stone fragmentation, facilitating passage.
  2. Renal stones less than 5 mm can usually pass spontaneously.
  3. Following formation of the first stone, patients should be advised to decrease calcium intake. Treatment of an underlying disease causing hypercalcemia should be considered.

- Struvite stones should be treated by management of the underlying infection. These stones also respond well to ESWL. If formation of a staghorn has occurred, percutaneus nephrostomy is required.
- Uric acid stones do not respond well to ESWL. Urine alkalization and aggressive hydration usually dissolve the stone. Patients should be advised to decrease protein intake, and maintain alkaline urine. Prophylaxis can be attained by use of allolpurinol.
- Cystine stones do not respond well to ESWL. Treatment consists of increasing urine output, alkalization, and reduction in protein intake (especially meat). Drug treatments are avoided if possible because of side affects.

RENAL MASSES

General
- Renal masses can be benign or malignant. Over 70% of renal masses are benign and cystic in nature.
- The most frequent type of malignancy of the kidney is metastatic disease.
- The most common primary tumor is renal cell carcinoma, which is twice as common in males. Renal cell carcinoma originates from the proximal convoluted tubules.
- Renal cell carcinoma commonly metastasizes to bones, the lungs and the brain, but metastasis may also occur to the contralateral kidney and liver.
- Transitional cell carcinoma is another type of cancer that may originate from the renal calyces or pelvis.

Clinical Manifestations and Management
- *CLASSIC PRESENTATION:* A patient who presents with hematuria, flank pain or tenderness, weight loss, anemia, and hypertension. A palpable mass may often be felt on physical examination.
- Cystic masses are asymptomatic.
- Hematuria is the most common symptom of renal cancer.
- Diagnostic modalities include urinalysis, IVP, ultrasound, and CT scan.
- A mass that appears cystic on ultrasound should have a FNA performed, which will differentiate benign from malignant.
- A mass that appears solid on ultrasound should be examined by CT scan, with surgery performed as necessary.
- Radical nephrectomy is indicated for renal cell carcinoma. Surgery should include excision of the adrenal, including Gerota's fascia.
- The prognosis of renal cell carcinoma depends on the stage of the cancer.
- If there is clinical suspicion of metastasis, further workup is indicated, including IVP, chest x-ray, liver function tests, and calcium levels.

NOTES

Chapter 7

NEUROLOGY

Theodore X. O'Connell, M.D.

HEADACHE

emorrhage

RESENTATION: A 35- to 65-year-old patient with the sudden onset of ... eadache of my life." The pain is often described as a "thunderclap" that is worst at the initial onset and may slowly improve.

- Subarachnoid hemorrhage is usually due to rupture of an intracerebral (berry) aneurysm, most commonly in the anterior part of the circle of Willis.
- Look for a history of other severe headaches suggesting warning leaks.
- There may be neurologic deficits present or an altered level of consciousness.
- Focal neurologic deficits result from vasospasm.
- Nausea, vomiting, and stiff neck may be present.
- Ruptured berry aneurysm is more common in females, patients with a history of coarctation of the aorta, and patients with polycystic kidney disease.
- Death may result from a recurrent hemorrhage, usually within 2 weeks of the first hemorrhage.
- Surgically repair by clipping the aneurysm.

Classic Migraine

- *CLASSIC PRESENTATION:* A female with unilateral and often retro-orbital throbbing headache with visual symptoms, photophobia, and nausea.
- Visual symptoms include flashing lights, colors, spots, or lines.
- The patient may have unilateral numbness, tingling, limb weakness, or confusion.
- Other symptoms include irritability and malaise.
- Attacks are recurrent.
- Onset is often in the teens and is more common in females.
- Migraines are exacerbated by stress, oral contraceptive pills, and menstruation.
- Treat with ergotamine with or without caffeine.

Common Migraine

- The presentation is similar to classic migraine, but without the prodromal aura.

Tumor

- *CLASSIC PRESENTATION:* A patient with intermittent pressure headaches that progress over many months and are worse with coughing, sneezing, or bending over.
- The headache is usually bilateral and constant rather than throbbing.
- There is a waxing and waning course to the headache. It may be worse in the morning or after lying down.
- Neurologic deficits may be present.

- Sudden exacerbation of the headache usually results from hemorrhage within the tumor or acute herniation.
- Death results from brain stem compression due to herniation with increased intracranial pressure.

Meningitis

- *CLASSIC PRESENTATION:* A patient with a severe headache accompanied by stiff neck, fever, photophobia, and focal infection.
- Signs of meningeal irritation include nuchal rigidity and a positive Brudzinski's sign (involuntary knee flexion during rapid neck flexion).
  For further details, see page 158 (Infections).

Tension Headache

- *CLASSIC PRESENTATION:* A patient with a bilateral, nonthrobbing, constant, dull aching headache usually described as having a pressing or tightening quality.
- The pain is continuous and is not aggravated by routine physical activities.
- There is no associated nausea and vomiting.
- Tension headache is usually accompanied by neck and trapezius muscle tenderness.

Cluster Headache

- *CLASSIC PRESENTATION:* A patient who presents with clusters of recurrent severe headaches described as a stabbing pain "deep behind the eye," interrupted by headache-free periods.
- Cluster headache is associated with tearing, facial flushing, rhinorrhea, and ptosis.
- The headaches are severe, but often of short duration.
- Cluster headaches are more common in men and are exacerbated by alcohol consumption.
- Treat with ergotamine with or without caffeine.

Sinus Headache

- *CLASSIC PRESENTATION:* A patient with a frontal headache associated with facial pain/tenderness and rhinorrhea.
- Sinus radiographs show mucosal thickening.
- Treat with decongestants, antihistamines, and antibiotics.
- Surgical drainage occasionally is necessary.

Temporal Arteritis (Giant Cell Arteritis)

- *CLASSIC PRESENTATION:* A patient over age 55 with a headache localized over the distribution of the temporal artery and associated with fever, malaise, visual symptoms, jaw claudication, and scalp tenderness.

- The features above are related to ischemia in the regions supplied by the carotid artery.
- The headache may be throbbing or nonthrobbing and unilateral or bilateral.
- Erythrocyte sedimentation rate (ESR) is increased.
- Half of all patients also have *polymyalgia rheumatica* (aching and stiffness of the shoulder and hip girdles).
- Patients require steroids early and in high doses to avoid blindness.
- Diagnosis requires confirmatory temporal artery biopsy that shows granulomatous inflammation.

Trigeminal Neuralgia

- *CLASSIC PRESENTATION:* A patient over age 40 with paroxysmal lancinating pain in the distribution of the trigeminal nerve.
- There is no associated weakness or sensory loss.
- Pain can be initiated by touching trigger points on the face.
- Trigeminal neuralgia is more common in females.
- Treat with carbamazepine.

Pseudotumor Cerebri (Benign Intracranial Hypertension)

- *CLASSIC PRESENTATION:* An obese female of child-bearing age with a nonthrobbing headache that is worse in the morning or with maneuvers that increase intracranial pressure (similar to headache due to tumor).
- Pseudotumor cerebri can be caused by vitamin A excess.
- It is associated with blurred vision progressing to blind spots and eventually vision loss.
- Papilledema may be seen on physical examination.
- Lumbar puncture shows normal CSF with very increased pressure.
- Treat with weight reduction, acetazolamide, and steroids.

STROKE

Stroke

- *CLASSIC PRESENTATION:* An older person with one or more rapidly developing focal neurologic deficit(s) persisting more than 24 hours.
- Stroke has a vascular etiology with brain tissue destruction secondary to hemorrhage or ischemia.
- Differentiate a stroke from a transient ischemic attack (TIA), which is a rapidly developing focal neurologic deficit resulting from ischemia, but which persists for less than 24 hours. There is only brain tissue dysfunction with no tissue destruction.

Risk Factors for Stroke

- Hypertension
- Transient ischemic attacks
- Coronary artery disease
- Congestive heart failure
- Diabetes mellitus
- Smoking
- Obesity
- Chronic atrial fibrillation
- Asymptomatic carotid bruits

Thromboembolic Stroke

- *CLASSIC PRESENTATION:* A person with a neurologic deficit(s) with a sudden onset and no warning; the deficit(s) is maximal at the onset.
- These strokes occur most often during waking hours.

Hemorrhagic Stroke

- *CLASSIC PRESENTATION:* A person with a gradually developing neurologic deficit(s) associated with headache, nausea, vomiting, and stiff neck. The individual often has a history of hypertension or bleeding disorder.
- These strokes also usually occur during waking hours.

Thrombotic Stroke

- *CLASSIC PRESENTATION:* A person with a prior history of transient ischemic attacks who has a neurologic deficit that develops in a stepwise fashion (sudden worsening, then stability, then further sudden worsening).
- These can evolve over several hours to days.
- Thrombotic strokes often occur overnight while the patient is sleeping and become evident upon awakening.

Lesion Localization

- TIAs that occur in the carotid distribution (cerebral hemispheres) commonly present with symptoms such as visual loss in one eye (amaurosis fugax), unilateral weakness, unilateral sensory disturbance, or language disturbances (aphasia).
- TIAs that occur in the vertebrobasilar distribution (brain stem or cerebellum) commonly present with symptoms such as vertigo, dizziness, ataxia, nausea, vomiting, dysphagia, sudden loss of consciousness, double vision (diplopia), or sensory disturbances in the face.

Diagnosis

- An EKG should be obtained to rule out a myocardial infarction or atrial fibrillation.
- A blood glucose level should be obtained because hypoglycemia and hyperglycemia can cause focal neurologic symptoms

INFECTIONS

Meningitis

- *CLASSIC PRESENTATION:* A patient with headache, fever, lethargy, confusion, stiff neck, nausea, vomiting, weakness, and/or photophobia.
- A petechial or purpuric rash may be seen over the trunk and extremities, in particular with meningococcal meningitis.
- Kernig's sign is resistance to knee extension after flexion of hips and knees.
- Brudzinski's sign is involuntary knee flexion during rapid neck flexion.
- Predisposing factors include bacteremia, chronic renal failure, immune system compromise, and disruption of protective barriers, such as with a basilar skull fracture.
- A CT scan should be done before lumbar puncture in patients with signs of increased intracranial pressure to avoid causing brainstem herniation.
- Normal CSF glucose levels are about 60% of blood glucose levels.
- CSF normally contains no neutrophils, so suspect bacterial meningitis if you see any neutrophils in the CSF.
- Steroids (e.g., dexamethasone) are often given to decrease inflammation.
- Antibiotic choice depends upon the etiologic agent, but empirically one of the broad-spectrum cephalosporins should be used (cefotaxime or ceftriaxone), as well as vancomycin if pneumococcal meningitis is suspected. The choice of antibiotic should be narrowed when the culture and sensitivity results come back from the laboratory.

Bacterial vs. Viral Meningitis

Characteristic	Bacterial	Viral
Opening pressure	Usually elevated	Normal to moderately elevated
CSF WBCs	100-1000, mostly PMNs	10-500, mostly lymphocytes
Protein	Elevated	Normal or slightly elevated
Glucose	Low	Normal
Misc.	Gram's stain + in about 60% of cases	

DEGENERATIVE DISEASES

Alzheimer's Disease
- *CLASSIC PRESENTATION:* A patient over age 65 with progressive dementia but no disturbance of consciousness.
- This is the most common cause of dementia.
- There must be an absence of systemic or other brain disease.
- Definitive diagnosis requires brain biopsy or autopsy.
- Neuropathic findings include neurofibrillary tangles and senile plaques.
- Clinical dementia with histopathologic findings of Alzheimer's disease occurs in virtually all patients with Down's syndrome who live past the age of 30.

Parkinson's Disease
- *CLASSIC PRESENTATION:* An older patient with the triad of resting tremor, rigidity, and bradykinesia.
- The resting tremor classically presents with a "pill-rolling" movement of the hands.
- Rigidity presents with the cogwheel phenomenon of the extremities on passive movement.
- Classically, the patient has bradykinesia with an immobile, expressionless face.
- Postural changes include stooped shoulders with neck, back, and knee flexion.
- Patients have difficulty initiating movement.
- This is an idiopathic progressive disorder of middle or late adult life that is caused by degeneration of the substantia nigra.
- Treat with L-dopa and carbidopa or anticholinergic agents such as benztropine.

Huntington's Disease

- *CLASSIC PRESENTATION:* A patient around the age of 35 with progressive choreoathetosis and dementia, frequently accompanied by depression.
- This is caused by an autosomal dominant mutation in a gene on chromosome 4.
- Atrophy of the caudate nucleus seen on CT scan is characteristic of Huntington's disease.

Multiple Sclerosis

- *CLASSIC PRESENTATION:* A 20- to 40-year-old woman with relapsing and remitting attacks of visual impairment, limb weakness, and diplopia that may progress to generalized weakness, spasticity, pain, swallowing difficulties, and dementia.
- This is the most common demyelinating disease of the CNS and is characterized by relapsing and remitting attacks involving multiple locations within the nervous system.
- Symptoms are often transient and fluctuate in severity.
- Symptoms may seem bizarre since they often are unable to be confirmed by the physical examiner.
- The patient may have sudden, electric shock-like, tingling paresthesias in the neck, which radiate into the arms during neck flexion.
- Late symptoms include generalized weakness, spasticity, pain, hearing loss, dysarthria, swallowing difficulties, and dementia.
- Optic neuritis may be visible on funduscopic examination and is associated with a loss of visual acuity.
- MRI shows multiple areas of white matter demyelination, especially in the periventricular regions.
- Abnormalities are seen on cortical evoked potentials.
- The clinical course is unpredictable and highly variable.
- The etiology is unknown, but is believed to result from both a genetic propensity and environmental factors.
- There is an unusual geographic distribution with an increasing frequency as the distance from the equator increases.
- There is no cure available, but immunosuppressive agents may be given to decrease exacerbations and extend periods of remission.

Central Pontine Myelinolysis

- *CLASSIC PRESENTATION:* An ICU patient with flaccid quadriplegia and facial and oropharyngeal weakness after having a rapid correction of hypernatremia.
- Central pontine myelinolysis can be prevented by correcting hypernatremia slowly.
- This is also seen in alcoholics and malnourished patients.

DISORDERS OF THE NEUROMUSCULAR JUNCTION

Myasthenia Gravis

- *CLASSIC PRESENTATION:* A young woman or older man with a complaint of double vision, difficulty swallowing and speaking, limb weakness and fatigue, especially after exercise.
- This is an autoimmune disorder caused by antibodies directed against the acetylcholine receptor at the neuromuscular junction.
- Peak incidence is in younger women, often in their 30s.
- It most severely affects the ocular muscles.
- Although many patients initially present with diplopia or ptosis, they eventually progress to more generalized head and neck muscle weakness and then finally extremity muscle weakness.
- The diagnosis can be made by giving a test dose of an acetylcholinesterase inhibitor (such as edrophonium), which results in transient dramatic improvement.
- Acetylcholine receptor antibodies can usually be detected in the blood.
- A CT scan or MRI may reveal the presence of a thymoma.
- Treat with a cholinesterase inhibitor (pyridostigmine).
- Thymectomy may lead to improvement.

Lambert-Eaton Syndrome

- *CLASSIC PRESENTATION:* An individual with a progressive generalized muscle weakness that improves with exercise.
- It is caused by antibodies directed against the calcium channels on the presynaptic membrane of the neuromuscular junction, resulting in interference with the release of acetylcholine vesicles.
- Lambert-Eaton myasthenic syndrome often is associated with small cell carcinoma of the lung.
- Proximal muscles are affected more than distal muscle groups.
- Absent tendon reflexes and mild sensory loss are present.
- The patient may have autonomic symptoms such as ptosis, impotence, dry mouth, and constipation.
- Treatment is directed at the underlying problem, though guanidine or immunosuppressive agents may be helpful.

BRAIN MASSES

Pituitary Adenoma

- *CLASSIC PRESENTATION:* An individual with bitemporal hemianopsia and headache with or without signs of acromegaly, Cushing's disease, or hyperprolactinemia.
- Bitemporal hemianopsia refers to vision loss in the superior temporal visual quadrants and is due to impingement on the optic chiasm.
- Increased growth hormone results in gigantism if it occurs before puberty and acromegaly if it occurs after puberty.
- Cushing's disease is due to excessive glucocorticoids and results in truncal obesity, hypertension, hirsutism, abdominal striae, and personality changes.
- Hyperprolactinemia results in galactorrhea and amenorrhea in women and impotence, decreased libido, and gynecomastia in men.
- Bromocriptine may be given to reduce prolactin levels.
- Treat the tumor with surgical resection.

Elevated Intracranial Pressure

- *CLASSIC PRESENTATION:* A patient with the following signs and symptoms: headache, nausea, vomiting, papilledema, and visual changes.
- Mechanisms of increased intracranial pressure include any of the following:
    1. Increased intracranial volume (tumor, hemorrhage, abscess).
    2. Acute brain swelling (anoxia, hypertensive encephalopathy, Reye's syndrome).
    3. High venous pressure (heart failure, superior vena cava syndrome).
    4. CSF flow obstruction.
- In children, the cranial sutures are not yet closed, so elevated intracranial pressure may be manifested by enlargement of the head or bulging fontanelles.
- Management includes the following:
    1. Elevate the patient's head to optimize venous drainage.
    2. Hyperventilate the patient, which decreases arterial pCO_2, resulting in cerebral vasoconstriction and consequent reduction in intracranial blood volume.
    3. Mannitol causes an osmotic fluid shift out of the brain.
    4. Glucocorticoids may decrease edema.

TRAUMA

Basilar Skull Fracture

- *CLASSIC PRESENTATION:* A patient with a history of head trauma who presents with Battle's sign and raccoon eyes. Also look for CSF otorrhea and rhinorrhea, and hemotympanum.
- Battle's sign is subcutaneous blood seen over the mastoid and is often associated with tympanic membrane rupture and blood or cerebrospinal fluid drainage into the middle ear.
- Raccoon eyes is the name for blood in the periorbital soft tissues and is often associated with CSF leakage into the sinuses.

Epidural Hematoma

- *CLASSIC PRESENTATION:* A patient with initial unconsciousness due to head trauma followed by a period of consciousness, then followed by progressive headache, drowsiness, hemiparesis, and a dilated pupil on the side of the hemorrhage.
- Epidural hematoma is caused by a tear of the middle meningeal artery.
- On CT scan a rapidly expanding mass is seen between the dura and cranial bone.
- This requires immediate neurosurgical evacuation of the clot.

Subdural Hematoma

- *CLASSIC PRESENTATION:* An elderly patient who has had a fall and presents with headache, confusion, hemiparesis, and lethargy.
- Subdural hematoma results from damage to bridging veins.
- Subdural hematoma is more common than an epidural hematoma since only minimal trauma is necessary to tear the veins.
- A subdural hematoma is a common complication of child abuse and is associated with retinal hemorrhages in the shaken baby syndrome.
- Subdural hematoma represents the accumulation of blood between arachnoid mater and dura mater.
- This requires neurosurgical drainage.
- An acute hemorrhage may mimic an epidural hematoma.

Concussion

- *CLASSIC PRESENTATION:* An individual with temporary impairment of brain function following head injury that results in a brief loss of consciousness.
- Patients may have impaired memory, poor concentration, blurred vision, tinnitus, dizziness, and nausea when they regain consciousness.

Spinal Cord Trauma

- The most common sites of injury are the lower cervical cord and the thoracolumbar junction.
- Spinal shock occurs initially with bilateral flaccid paralysis and sensory loss below the level of the lesion.
- It may also be accompanied by areflexia and bladder and bowel dysfunction.
- After several weeks there may be slow recovery with increased reflex activity below the level of the lesion.
- Autonomic disturbances include profuse sweating, orthostatic hypotension, and bladder dysfunction.
- The Brown-Séquard syndrome (cord hemisection) involves ipsilateral spastic weakness, ipsilateral loss of proprioception, and contralateral loss of pain and temperature sensation.
- Management includes immobilization of the neck and back, corticosteroids in high dosage, and radiologic films to determine the site and extent of injury.

Chapter 8

PSYCHIATRY

Susan L. Taylor, M.D.
and
Theodore X. O'Connell, M.D.

MOOD DISORDERS

Major Depression

- *CLASSIC PRESENTATION:* A patient of any age who presents with depressed mood or anhedonia (loss of interest or pleasure) and other symptoms including significant weight loss or gain, insomnia or hypersomnia, psychomotor agitation or retardation, fatigue or loss of energy, feelings of worthlessness or guilt, suicidal ideations, difficulty thinking or concentrating, and/or recurrent thoughts of death.
- The patient's symptoms cause significant distress or impaired functioning. The symptoms are not accounted for by the effects of a substance or medication, nor by recent bereavement. The symptoms persist for longer than 2 months.
- Pseudodementia is a state clinically identical to irreversible senile dementia but is not caused by an organic condition. It is a form of depression that often resolves with antidepressant medications.
- The lifetime prevalence of depression is 9% to 20%.
- First-degree relatives of depressed people have a 2 to 3 times increased risk over the general population.
- The principal treatment for depression is antidepressants. Drug selection is based on the patient's general medical condition, the drug's side effects, and a personal or family history of therapeutic response to a specific agent.
- About 70% of patients respond favorably to antidepressants. Psychosocial therapies are also often used.

Dysthymic Disorder

- *CLASSIC PRESENTATION:* A patient who presents with chronically depressed mood for at least 2 years. The patient has had no major depressive episodes or manic episodes but has chronic feelings of inadequacy and loss of interest or pleasure in most activities of daily life. The depressive symptoms are usually mild or moderate.
- Think of dysthymic disorder as a mild form of depressive disorder.
- Depressive symptoms include poor appetite, overeating, sleep problems, fatigue, feelings of hopelessness, low self-esteem, and poor concentration.
- Dysthymic disorder occurs more often in individuals with a history of long-term stress and sudden emotional loss.
- Symptoms often worsen later in the day.
- This disorder is more prevalent in women and generally occurs in people in their 20s or 30s.
- The principal treatment is psychotherapy. Many patients may also benefit from a trial of antidepressants or lithium.

Bipolar Disorder
- *CLASSIC PRESENTATION:* A young patient who presents with a past or present history of manic episodes cycling with a depressed state. The manic episodes are characterized by a predominantly elevated, expansive, or irritable mood.
- The manic episodes are characterized by feelings of abundant energy, decreased need for sleep, rapid speech, and euphoria. The patient may stop conforming to social norms.
- The peak age of onset is 20 to 25 years.
- The prognosis is usually good.
- There is clearly a strong genetic component. The concordance rate in monozygotic twins is 65% to 85%.
- Lithium is the treatment of choice for the acute manic state. Alternative medicines include carbamazepine and valproate.
- Psychosocial intervention also is often needed.

Cyclothymic Disorder
- *CLASSIC PRESENTATION:* A female who presents with manic and depressive states that are not of sufficient duration or severity to be considered bipolar disorder. The symptoms have persisted for more than 2 years and have no psychotic component.
- Cyclothymic disorder is characterized by short cycles of depression and hypomania.

ANXIETY DISORDERS

Generalized Anxiety Disorder
- *CLASSIC PRESENTATION:* A patient who presents with excessive anxiety and worry about a number of events or activities. The worry is difficult for the person to control and causes impairment in daily functioning.
- Symptoms include restlessness, feeling easily fatigued, difficulty concentrating, irritability, muscle tension, and sleep disturbances.
- Generalized anxiety disorder usually causes less dysfunction than other anxiety disorders.
- Treat with benzodiazepines or tricyclic antidepressants.

Panic Disorder
- *CLASSIC PRESENTATION:* A young female college student who comes to see her doctor after she experienced a discrete period of intense fear or discomfort that was accompanied by symptoms such as palpitations, sweating, trembling, sensation of shortness of breath, chest pain, nausea, dizziness, and/or fear of dying.
- Patients often have recurrent unexpected panic attacks with persistent concern about having additional attacks.

- The attacks generally begin suddenly and resolve in about 10 minutes.
- Caffeine, alcohol, and marijuana are frequent causes of anxiety symptoms. Similar symptoms may also be provoked by cold medications, thyroid hormone, digitalis, and stimulants.
- Peak age of onset is 15 to 25 years.
- Treat with antidepressants.

Posttraumatic Stress Disorder (PTSD)

- *CLASSIC PRESENTATION:* A patient with a history of significant psychological trauma or stress in his or her life who presents with substantial disruption in their normal level of functioning. The suffering is frequently associated with re-experiencing the trauma in thoughts or dreams, persistent symptoms of arousal, and signs of numbing or avoidance.
- Symptoms persist for at least 1 month.
- PTSD must be differentiated from an adjustment disorder.
- Acute PTSD usually responds well to supportive measures with return to normal activity if support is promptly given after the traumatic event.
- Patients with acute PTSD do best if they are allowed to talk about their experiences and encouraged to return to normal activities as quickly as possible.
- Chronic PTSD may last for decades with varying degrees of disability.

Agoraphobia

- *CLASSIC PRESENTATION:* A patient with a fear of being caught in a situation in which quick escape would be difficult or embarrassing. Patients are often fearful of going out in public (eating out, auditoriums, shopping).
- These patients often describe situations in which they would feel trapped. They often have a fear of panic, fainting, or dying.
- Most patients recognize the irrationality of their fears and lament their inability to face everyday situations.
- Patients have anticipatory anxiety about being caught in fearful situations.
- Exposure therapy may be effective.

Other Phobias

- Social phobia is the persistent irrational fear of embarrassment when performing in social situations. The person recognizes that the fear is excessive or unreasonable.
- The avoidance of social situations or distress in the situation interferes with occupational, social, or relationship functioning.
- Social phobias are treated with β-blockers.
- Common specific phobias are irrational fear of snakes, spiders, heights, small closed spaces, and flying.
- Exposure to the specific phobic stimulus usually provokes an immediate anxiety response.

- The patient recognizes that the fear is excessive or unreasonable.
- Treat with exposure therapy.

Obsessive-Compulsive Disorder

- *CLASSIC PRESENTATION:* A patient usually presents with obsessions (repetitive intrusive ideas, images, or impulses) and compulsions (repetitive thoughts or acts performed to decrease anxiety or discomfort associated with obsessions).
- Attempts are usually made to resist these rituals. However, if they are prevented from carrying out a ritual, obsessive-compulsive individuals become anxious.
- The behaviors or mental acts are aimed at preventing or reducing distress or preventing some dreaded event.
- The person recognizes that the obsession is the product of his or her own mind and is not imposed from without.
- They recognize that the obsessions and compulsions are excessive or unreasonable, are time-consuming, and interfere with daily functioning.
- Obsessive-compulsive disorder clusters in families.
- Treatment consists of selective serotonin reuptake inhibitors or clomipramine as well as behavioral therapy.

DELIRIUM AND DEMENTIA

Delirium

- *CLASSIC PRESENTATION:* A patient of any age who presents in a stuporous state with impaired ability to focus or sustain attention. His family states that he previously acted normally and was completely alert. He is found to be disoriented, and his speech is incoherent.
- Delirium is a disturbance of consciousness.
- Patients with delirium perform poorly on tests of attention and commonly also have memory deficits.
- Patients with delirium also have a change in cognition, often accompanied by perceptual disturbances such as visual hallucinations.
- The disturbance develops over a short period of time, usually hours to days.
- One of the most significant aspects of delirium is that the course usually fluctuates, with patients alternating from stuporous to agitated over the course of a given day.
- Delirium can be caused by medical conditions (e.g., metabolic imbalance), substance abuse, drug toxicity, withdrawal, head trauma, infection, etc.
- Delirium is treated by treating the causative factors.

Dementia

- *CLASSIC PRESENTATION:* An elderly woman is brought in by her family for "problems with her memory." Her family states that over the past few years she has become more forgetful. She sometimes forgets the name of her own daughter, and recently when she went to the grocery store she could not find her way home. However, when asked anything about her husband, who passed away 10 years ago, she can answer the question with great detail.

- Dementia is characterized by multiple cognitive deficits with memory impairment. Recent memory usually is more affected than remote memory.
- Cognitive deficits may include impaired language skills, difficulty with abstract thinking, and inability to identify or recognize objects.
- Grooming and hygiene may be impaired.
- Mood is commonly depressed.
- Dementia usually has a very gradual onset, and the course of this illness may be progressive, static, or remitting.
- Dementia is found predominantly in the elderly.
- Dementia may be the result of Alzheimer's disease, vascular causes, may be secondary to another medical condition, or may be substance-induced.
- Alzheimer's type dementia is the most common cause of dementia.
- Treat the underlying cause, if possible.

Comparison of Delirium and Dementia

Delirium	Dementia
Widely fluctuating course	Slow, progressive, worsening course
Acute (sudden) onset	Gradual onset
Hallucinations are common	Usually no hallucinations
Decreased level of consciousness	Normal level of consciousness
Impaired attention	Normal attention

Amnestic Disorder

- *CLASSIC PRESENTATION:* A patient who is unable to remember recent events that occurred after he was involved in an accident in which he suffered significant head trauma.
- Amnestic disorder is characterized by the development of memory impairment with the inability to learn new information or recall old information. This is a deficit in memory and new learning.
- Amnestic disorder can be caused by any insult to the brain.
- In anterograde amnesia, the patient is unable to recall recent events that have occurred since the damage to the brain.

- In retrograde amnesia, the patient cannot recall events that occurred before the insult to the brain.

PSYCHOTIC DISORDERS

Schizophrenia

- *CLASSIC PRESENTATION:* A 19-year-old male patient is referred to a psychiatrist because his primary care physician noticed that he had recently developed a flat affect and had informed his doctor that yesterday a celebrity told him from his television that he had the power to read other people's minds. Symptoms persist for more than 6 months.
- Schizophrenia is a severe and prolonged mental disturbance manifested by disturbed thought, speech, and behavior. Characteristic symptoms are hallucinations, delusions, bizarre behavior, and deterioration of general functioning.
- Schizophrenia usually presents in the second to third decade of life, and the onset is usually gradual over weeks to months. There is commonly a trigger event, and patients may have a prodrome of depression, anxiety, suspiciousness, hypochondriasis, and difficulty concentrating. Patients usually have a gradual withdrawal from people and activities.
- There is clearly a genetic component in the predisposition to schizophrenia.
- Characteristic disturbances include:
    1. Language and communication (problems with train of thought, incoherency).
    2. Content of thought.
        a. Delusions or false beliefs (thought broadcasting and thought insertion).
        b. Patients may feel that TV or newspapers have personal messages for them.
        c. Patients may have delusions of having special powers.
    3. Disturbances in perception e.g., hallucinations, most commonly auditory.
    4. Altered affect which may be inappropriate, labile, or flattened. Patients may report that they are "losing their feelings."
    5. Changes in sense of self e.g., patients can have doubts and worries about their identity.
    6. Volition, e.g., patients have a loss of goal-directed activity that may impair work performance.
- Positive and Negative Symptoms of Schizophrenia

Positive Symptoms	Negative Symptoms
Hallucinations, delusions, bizarre behavior, disorganized speech seen early in the course of the disease	Emotional blunting, social withdrawal, cognitive deficits associated with family history of schizophrenia indicate poor prognosis
Usually suppressed by neuroleptics	Less favorable response to neuroleptics

- Neuroleptic medications control acute symptoms, decrease hospital stays, and prolong remission.

Schizophreniform Disorder

- *CLASSIC PRESENTATION:* Similar to schizophrenia, but the person returns to their previous level of functioning within 6 months.
- Schizophreniform disorder is a psychotic illness with symptoms typical of schizophrenia, but it is not as chronic as schizophrenia.
- Schizophreniform disorder is less common than schizophrenia and the etiology is unknown.
- Treatment: Most patients require neuroleptic drugs.

Schizoaffective Disorder

- *CLASSIC PRESENTATION:* A patient who presents with psychotic symptoms consistent with schizophrenia, but these symptoms are often accompanied by manic or depressive symptoms.
- Most commonly seen in young adulthood.
- Treatment includes neuroleptics to control psychotic symptoms, lithium for manic symptoms, and antidepressants for depressive symptoms.

Delusional Disorder

- *CLASSIC PRESENTATION:* A patient who presents with prominent, well-organized delusions (but no hallucinations), abnormal affect, and disorganized thought and behavior.
- These delusions become the focus of the patient's life.
- This is a relatively uncommon disorder, with the onset usually in middle age or older.
- Treatment is with neuroleptics.

Brief Psychotic Disorder

- *CLASSIC PRESENTATION:* A patient who presents with delusions, hallucinations, and/or disorganized speech or behavior for at least 1 day and less than 1 month.

- This disorder is often preceded by a stressful event. Brief psychotic disorder also can occur postpartum.
- There is always a full recovery.

SUBSTANCE-RELATED DISORDERS

Substance Abuse
- Substance abuse is defined as the use of a substance, resulting in failure to fulfill obligations at home, work, or school.
- There may be a history of a DUI, arrests, fights, and other antisocial behavior.
- This is different from substance dependence because there is no tolerance or withdrawal.

Substance Dependence
- *CLASSIC PRESENTATION:* A patient with a maladaptive pattern of substance use (e.g., alcohol) leading to clinically significant impairment or distress.
- This disorder is characterized by:
    1. Tolerance (need to increase amounts of a substance to reach a desired effect).
    2. Withdrawal (development of a substance-specific syndrome due to decreased substance intake).
    3. Alteration in social or occupational activities.
    4. Spending significant time seeking, using, or recovering from use of a substance

Stimulants
- *CLASSIC PRESENTATION:* The patient is agitated, tachycardic, and hypertensive, and has a history of recent insomnia. The pupils are found to be dilated on physical examination.
- The 2 most prevalent stimulants are nicotine and caffeine.
- Cocaine use causes euphoria followed by depression.
- Major stimulants of abuse are cocaine and amphetamines.
- Cocaine users may have seizures, hypertensive crises, or cerebrovascular accidents.
- Withdrawal symptoms include cravings, hypersomnolence, and depression.
- Treat psychosis with haloperidol and give tricyclic antidepressants to decrease cravings.

Phencyclidine (PCP) Intoxication
- *CLASSIC PRESENTATION:* A patient who is hostile, paranoid, and who may describe a clouded sensorium.
- PCP is used for mind-altering experiences and to cause euphoria.

- Patients using PCP may have hypertension, seizures, psychosis, agitation, respiratory depression, or coma.
- Treat violence with haloperidol and seizures with benzodiazepines.

Barbiturates
- *CLASSIC PRESENTATION:* A patient with slurred speech, altered gait, nystagmus, lethargy, respiratory depression, and/or coma. On physical examination the pupils are constricted, and the patient is hypotensive and diaphoretic with a decreased respiratory rate.
- Intoxication causes sedation, euphoria, and analgesia.
- Treat barbiturate overdose with emesis, gastric lavage, and urinary alkalinization.

Benzodiazepines
- *CLASSIC PRESENTATION:* A patient may present in withdrawal psychosis, sometimes with seizures.
- Treat with phenobarbital.
- Benzodiazepines are very widely used in the U.S., often as sleep-aids and for anxiety relief.

Marijuana
- *CLASSIC PRESENTATION:* A patient may complain of mild withdrawal symptoms such as insomnia, anxiety, perspiration, and/or upset stomach.
- Heavy use compromises pulmonary function and suppresses testosterone.

Opiates
- *CLASSIC PRESENTATION:* A patient who has taken an overdose of opiates presents with pinpoint pupils, respiratory depression, flushed warm skin, and a declining level of consciousness. It may progress to shock, hypotension, and coma.
- Opiates are used as analgesics but are also used illicitly for euphoria and "escape". Opiate use causes sedation, euphoria, and hypoactivity.
- Adverse effects are drowsiness and nausea.
- Withdrawal symptoms include mydriasis, sweating, and cravings.
- Treat overdose with naloxone (opiate antagonist). Decrease withdrawal symptoms with clonidine.

Alcohol
- *CLASSIC PRESENTATION:* A patient who presents with ataxia, slurred speech, disinhibitory behavior, and difficulty thinking and/or concentrating may be intoxicated from alcohol. Overdose can present with severe respiratory depression, coma, and death.

- An alcoholic frequently denies or grossly underestimates his own consumption of alcohol. He frequently lies to his family, friends, and physicians about his dependence on alcohol and continues to drink despite adverse effects on other areas of his life.
- The lifetime prevalence of alcoholism is approximately 5 times higher in men than in women.
- There is a hereditary component for alcoholism.
- Withdrawal can cause delirium tremens and seizures.
- Prevent delirium tremens with benzodiazepines.
- The physician can attempt to treat with disulfiram, but most prefer to use treatment centers and/or AA groups due to the horrible nausea and vomiting caused by alcohol consumption when taking disulfiram.

SOMATOFORM DISORDERS

Somatization Disorder
- *CLASSIC PRESENTATION:* A patient with multiple physical symptoms that recur over a period of several years and are apparently unrelated to an identifiable physical disorder. The patient's physical complaints often are grossly exaggerated.
- Patients often self-medicate, seek medical attention, and/or change their lifestyles based on their physical symptoms.
- Anxiety and depressed mood are commonly associated symptoms.
- Physicians must rule out organic diseases, schizophrenia, depression, and panic disorders.
- There is an increased prevalence in women, and there is also a strong familial tendency.

Conversion Disorder
- *CLASSIC PRESENTATION:* A patient who presents with paralysis that is unusual in distribution, and cannot be explained by any known neurological disorder.
- Conversion disorder is characterized by the involuntary loss or alteration of physical functioning that can't be explained by any physical disorder.
- Neurological symptoms are most common, such as paralysis, blindness, and seizures.

Somatoform Pain Disorder
- *CLASSIC PRESENTATION:* A patient who has been seen by the physician many times over at least 6 months for complaints of pain in the absence of explanatory findings on physical examination.
- This is associated with an increased incidence of substance abuse.
- Patients with somatoform pain disorder may respond to antidepressants.

Hypochondriasis
- *CLASSIC PRESENTATION:* A patient who persistently seeks medical care for minor physical problems, and fears having or believes that they have a serious illness without any evidence of such.
- These patients often use many over-the-counter medicines.
- Associated with depression and anxiety.

Dissociative Disorder
- *CLASSIC PRESENTATION:* A patient who has had a sudden, temporary disruption of some aspect of consciousness, identity, or motor behavior.
- These are very uncommon but present with dramatic clinical pictures.
- Multiple personality disorder is a dissociative disorder, as is dissociative amnesia, which is memory loss following a stressful or traumatic life experience.
- Treatment often consists of psychotherapy. Barbiturates (amobarbital) may be useful in dissociative amnesia.

Adjustment Disorder
- *CLASSIC PRESENTATION:* A patient who develops emotional or behavioral symptoms in response to an identifiable stressor(s) occurring within 3 months of the identifiable stressor.
- Symptoms (disruption of social or occupational functioning) are in excess of those normally expected. The symptoms remit if the stressor ceases.
- Common in adolescents, this disorder is a disruption of the normal process of adaptation to stressful events.
- Treat with brief psychosocial intervention.

Factitious Disorder
- *CLASSIC PRESENTATION:* A patient who presents with psychological or physical symptoms that are deliberately and consciously simulated by the patient. The patient may be noted to not have symptoms when medical personnel are out of the room.
- There may be psychological symptoms such as delusions and hallucinations, or physical symptoms such as pain.
- This disorder is known as Munchausen syndrome when the symptoms are accompanied by physical signs.
- There is a greater incidence in men.
- Symptoms are voluntary, without unconscious or symbolic factors.

Malingering
- The presentation is the same as for factitious disorder, but malingerers have specific goals with obvious secondary gain, e.g., insurance payments, avoidance of work or avoidance of a jail term.

PERSONALITY DISORDERS

Paranoid Personality Disorder

- *CLASSIC PRESENTATION:* A person who has a pervasive distrust and suspiciousness of others, and believes that other people's motives are evil or malevolent. The patient may believe that people are "out to get him," or that there is a big conspiracy against him personally.
- Paranoid personality disorder is characterized by a suspicion, without evidence, that others are exploiting or harming the patient.
- People with this disorder are often distrustful, hostile, stubborn, defensive, and avoid intimacy.
- There is an increased incidence of paranoid personality disorder in men.

Schizoid Personality Disorder

- *CLASSIC PRESENTATION:* A person with an isolated lifestyle seemingly without longing for the companionship of others.
- These patients have a history of repeated episodes of detachment from social relationships and little or no expression of emotions in their interpersonal relations.
- They do not want to be close to others and choose solitude without feelings of loneliness. They have little interest in activities, including sexual relations.
- These people usually have few or no close friends and are described as emotionally cold and detached.

Schizotypal Personality Disorder

- *CLASSIC PRESENTATION:* A person who feels uncomfortable with and has had a lack of close relationships, and also has multiple oddities and eccentricities of manners, behavior, thought, speech, appearance, and affect.
- It is the eccentricities that differentiates schizotypal from schizoid personality disorder.
- About 10% of these patients commit suicide.
- Treatment is similar to that for schizophrenia.

Histrionic Personality Disorder

- *CLASSIC PRESENTATION:* A person with excessive emotionality and attention-seeking behavior. The patient often tries to draw attention to herself with dramatic, lively, and sometimes inappropriate sexually seductive or provocative behavior.
- The patient has rapidly shifting emotions, and considers relationships to be more intimate than they actually are.
- Persons with this disorder have a tendency toward somatization, with dramatic and changing physical symptoms.

Narcissistic Personality Disorder

- *CLASSIC PRESENTATION:* An arrogant person with haughty behaviors and attitudes who is very grandiose, has a sense of self-importance, lack of empathy for others, and constant need for admiration.
- Persons with this disorder believe themselves to be "special" and unique.
- This disorder is characterized by a preoccupation with fantasies of success, power, brilliance, beauty, or love.

Antisocial Personality Disorder

- *CLASSIC PRESENTATION:* A person with blatant disregard for and violation of the rights of others.
- This disorder is usually characterized by illegal, reckless, and impulsive behavior without remorse.
- Patients with this disorder are often described as deceitful, lying, irritable, and aggressive.
- Antisocial personality disorder may be diagnosed in up to 75% of prison inmates.
- There is an increased incidence of sociopathic behavior and alcoholism in the parents of patients with antisocial personality disorder, as well as a history of maternal deprivation.
- There is usually a history of conduct disorder as a child.

Borderline Personality Disorder

- *CLASSIC PRESENTATION:* Think *Fatal Attraction*: a person with a history of unstable interpersonal relationships, self-image, and affects. They are often described as very impulsive with rapid changes of goals and values, with often inappropriate, intense behavior.
- These patients are often preoccupied with threats of real or imagined abandonment, and are very needy in their interpersonal relationships.
- Persons with this disorder have an increased incidence of substance abuse, gambling addictions, unsafe sex and promiscuity, and recklessness.
- They may have recurrent suicidal threats or behavior, or self-mutilating behavior.

Avoidant Personality Disorder

- *CLASSIC PRESENTATION:* An intensely shy person with social inhibition who frequently feels inadequate and is hypersensitive to any type of criticism or rejection.
- These patients are very insecure.
- This patient avoids significant interpersonal contact for fear of rejection or criticism and views self as socially inept or inferior to others.

Dependent Personality Disorder

- *CLASSIC PRESENTATION:* A clingy person with excessive fear of separation and a constant need to be taken care of. The patient usually is submissive and has trouble taking responsibility for major areas in his life.
- These patients need excessive support and reassurance from others to make any kind of decision.
- They have difficulty expressing disagreement with others or doing things on their own.

Obsessive-Compulsive Personality Disorder

- *CLASSIC PRESENTATION:* A person who is preoccupied with neatness, perfectionism, and control. The patient is usually distressed with any indecisiveness and is generally inflexible.
- These patients have difficulty expressing tender feelings and are excessively devoted to work and productivity to the exclusion of leisure activities and friendships.
- They are usually rigid and stubborn and are often reluctant to delegate tasks or to work with others unless they submit to his way of doing things.
- A patient with obsessive-compulsive personality disorder does not have true obsessions or compulsions, as those with obsessive-compulsive disorder do.

CHILD PSYCHIATRY

Attention-Deficit/Hyperactivity Disorder (ADHD)

- *CLASSIC PRESENTATION:* A school-aged boy with motor overactivity, impulsivity, distractibility, and inattentiveness.
- Prevalence is about 3 to 5% and is more common in boys.
- Treat with stimulants like methylphenidate, dextroamphetamine, and pemoline. These medications reduce symptoms in about 75% of children.

Conduct Disorder

- *CLASSIC PRESENTATION:* A boy with an early history of aggressive behavior and violence against people and animals. He seems to be unable to follow social norms, and often will lie, cheat, and steal. There frequently is a history of torturing animals.
- These children often have antisocial personality disorder as adults.
- This disorder is associated with family instability, physical and sexual abuse, and family alcoholism.
- Treat with lithium or haloperidol, and psychological therapy.

Oppositional Defiant Disorder

- *CLASSIC PRESENTATION:* A child with negative, hostile, and defiant behavior who often loses his or her temper and argues with adults.
- Children with this disorder blame others for their mistakes.
- These children usually are not violent, in comparison to conduct disorder.
- Oppositional defiant disorder often occurs in families with overly rigid parents. This disorder appears to result from parent-child struggles over autonomy.
- Treat with family therapy.

Tourette's Disorder

- *CLASSIC PRESENTATION:* A 7- or 8-year-old boy with motor and vocal tics, such as repetitive eye blinking, facial grimacing, grunting, hitting, coprolalia (use of vulgar words), or echolalia (repeating others' words).
- Treat with haloperidol.

Autistic Disorder

- *CLASSIC PRESENTATION:* A child with an early history of difficulty with attachment to parents, impaired social interactions, impaired and/or late communication, and a restricted repertoire of behaviors and interests.
- Children with autistic disorder can be high or low functioning depending on IQ (70% have IQ < 70), communication skills, and severity of other symptoms.
- Asperger's disorder is characterized by autistic behavior without delays in language or cognitive development.
- Rett's disorder is a neurodegenerative disorder that affects girls only, who start out with normal development and become progressively worse.
- Treat autistic children with special education, family psychotherapy, and support. Haloperidol is sometimes used.

Separation Anxiety Disorder

- *CLASSIC PRESENTATION:* A child with excessive distress lasting greater than one month concerning separation from home or parents.
- These children often have recurrent nightmares and physical symptoms such as abdominal pain and vomiting.
- There is often a history of school avoidance.
- Treat with psychotherapy and imipramine.

Elimination Disorders

- Elimination disorders include encopresis (fecal incontinence) and enuresis (bedwetting).
- Physical disorders such as Hirschsprung's disease or urinary tract disorders should be ruled out before a diagnosis of an elimination disorder is made.

- Inadequate toilet training can result in child-parent power struggles and functional encopresis.
- Treat with behavior therapy and family guidance. Imipramine is often effective for enuresis.

Child Abuse and Neglect
- An estimated 1 million children are abused or neglected annually in the U.S.
- Risk factors for child abuse include low birth weight or premature infants, a disabled child, defiancy, or hyperactivity.
- In sexual abuse cases, 50% of the time the offender is a parent, parent surrogate, or relative.

EATING DISORDERS

Anorexia Nervosa
- *CLASSIC PRESENTATION:* An adolescent girl, involved in ballet or modeling, whose body weight is less than 85% of the ideal body weight, who refuses to maintain or gain weight due to an intense fear of becoming fat, even though she is underweight. The patient may present to a physician for amenorrhea.
- Anorexia nervosa is characterized by a disturbed body image.
- Treat as an inpatient if weight loss is extensive or if the patient refuses to eat or take medicine.
- Cyproheptadine and antidepressants may be helpful. Patients need cognitive behavior therapy aimed at changing their attitudes about eating and body image.

Bulimia Nervosa
- *CLASSIC PRESENTATION:* An adolescent girl who has had episodic, uncontrolled, and compulsive ingestion of large amounts of food over a short period of time (binge eating), followed by self-induced vomiting, use of laxatives or diuretics, fasting, or vigorous exercise in order to prevent weight gain (purging). On physical examination, she may have decaying teeth and calluses on her index and middle fingers.
- The decaying teeth are due to the effects of regurgitated stomach acid. The calluses are due to the fingers rubbing on the front teeth during self-induced vomiting.
- These patients do not usually have weight loss of more than 15% of body weight.
- These patients, like those with anorexia nervosa, also have a disturbed body image and cannot control their eating behaviors.
- Treatment is similar to that for anorexia.

SUICIDE

Suicide
- Successful suicide is 3 times more common in men and increases with advancing age. However, women have more suicide attempts. Men usually use more violent means.
- Guns are the most common means of successful suicide.
- Suicide is more common in single people.
- Patients at high risk for suicide are those patients with a plan, or who are intoxicated, unemployed, or poor.

PSYCHIATRIC MEDICATIONS

Antidepressants
- Tricyclic antidepressants (TCAs) inhibit reuptake of both norepinephrine and serotonin. They generally have similar efficacy, and the onset of antidepressant effects may take several weeks. TCAs can have many side effects including:
    1. Anticholinergic effects - dry mouth, blurred vision, urinary retention, and constipation
    2. Antihistamine effects - sedation
    3. Serotonergic effects - restlessness or sedation
    4. Adrenergic effects - tremor, excitement, palpitations, orthostatic hypotension, and weight gain
- Monoamine oxidase inhibitors (MAOIs) are used to treat atypical depression that is characterized by hypersomnia, hyperphagia, somatic complaints, and dysphoria. Common side effects include:
    1. Anticholinergic effects
    2. Sedation
    3. Orthostatic hypotension
    4. Hypertensive crisis with tyramine-containing foods including beer and red wine, cheeses and fava beans, as well as with all sympathomimetic amines such as over-the-counter cold remedies containing pseudoephedrine. MAOIs should be discontinued three weeks before surgery.
- Selective serotonin reuptake inhibitors (SSRIs) have a lower incidence of side effects, but common side effects include insomnia, psychomotor agitation, sexual dysfunction, tremor, headache, and occasionally nausea and diarrhea.
- Trazodone is a phenylpiperazine antidepressant that is a serotonin receptor blocker. Its major side effects are:
    1. Cardiac arrhythmia
    2. Dizziness

3.   Sedation
4.   Orthostatic hypotension
5.   Priapism - abnormal prolonged painful penile erections

Mood Stabilizers
● Lithium is the drug of choice for treating acute manic episodes and preventing manic recurrences. Side effects include:
1.   Dry mouth
2.   Urinary frequency
3.   Hypothyroidism and nontoxic goiter
4.   Nephrogenic diabetes insipidus
5.   Tremor
6.   Gastrointestinal distress
● Lithium has a low therapeutic index and lithium blood levels need to be monitored during treatment. Signs and symptoms of lithium toxicity include:
1.   Drowsiness and slurred speech
2.   Ataxia
3.   Hyperactive deep tendon reflexes
4.   Cardiac arrhythmias
5.   Seizures
● Carbamazepine and valproic acid are usually second-line agents used to treat mania.

Antipsychotics/Neuroleptics
● These drugs are used to treat schizophrenia, delusional disorder, brief psychotic episodes, and acute psychosis.
● All of the antipsychotics are about equal in efficacy and work by blocking dopamine receptors.
● Antipsychotics are either described as high-potency (haloperidol and fluphenazine) or low-potency (chlorpromazine, thioridazine, clozapine).
● Antipsychotics mainly decrease "positive symptoms" of psychosis such as hallucinations, delusions, thought disorder, and uncooperativeness.
● "Negative symptoms" such as flattened affect, anhedonia, apathy, and social withdrawal are less responsive to these drugs.
● High-potency neuroleptics have less sedation, hypotension, and anticholinergic side effects than low-potency neuroleptics. However, high-potency neuroleptics have an increased incidence of extrapyramidal side effects and neuroleptic malignant syndrome.
● Extrapyramidal side effects include:
1.   Acute dystonia - muscle spasms of the neck, face, mouth, and tongue (torticollis). This usually starts within days of initiating treatment. Treat by switching to a different neuroleptic.
2.   Akathisia - purposeless movements, usually of the legs, associated with a feeling of restlessness. Treat with anticholinergics.

3. Pseudoparkinsonism - resembles Parkinson's disease with cogwheeling movements, pill-rolling tremors, flat facies, and gait disturbances. Treat with anticholinergics and discontinuation of the current neuroleptic.
4. Tardive dyskinesia – a usually irreversible disorder characterized by lip smacking, tongue movements, and choreiform movements of the trunk and limbs, which occur during or after long-term use of antipsychotics. Treat by switching to a different antipsychotic.

- Neuroleptic malignant syndrome is a rare, life-threatening side effect of neuroleptics (more commonly high-potency), which is characterized by unexplained fevers, rigidity, pulmonary complications, and organ failure.
    1. It usually occurs after starting or increasing the dose of antipsychotics.
    2. Dantrolene is the treatment of choice. Bromocriptine can also be used.
- Clozapine is an atypical antipsychotic with an uncommon side effect of agranulocytosis.

Anxiolytics
- Benzodiazepines are used to treat panic attacks, generalized anxiety disorder, and are also used as sedatives. They produce physical dependence and tolerance. Side effects include sedation, dizziness, weakness, anterograde amnesia, ataxia, and falling. Withdrawal symptoms include anxiety, tremor, palpitations, sweating, nausea, confusion, and seizures. Withdraw benzodiazepines slowly.
- Buspirone is an anxiolytic that is unrelated to the benzodiazepines but is about equal in efficacy. It causes no sedation, tolerance, or withdrawal and has a low potential for abuse. Adverse effects include dizziness, nausea, headache, nervousness, lightheadedness, and excitement.

Chapter 9

DERMATOLOGY

Theodore X. O'Connell, M.D.

INFLAMMATORY DISORDERS

Contact Dermatitis
- *CLASSIC PRESENTATION:* A patient with erythema, papules, and pruritis on a body surface that follows a contact distribution.
- Typical areas of dermatitis are a waistband or bra strap distribution.
- An earlobe or "jewelry distribution" is typical of nickel allergy.
- The dermatitis may be caused by either chemical irritation or an allergic reaction.
- Treat by removing the offending agent and giving topical corticosteroids. In cases of nickel allergy, the patient should be instructed not to wear any jewelry that could contain nickel.

Rosacea
- *CLASSIC PRESENTATION:* A person with a long history of flushing and increased skin temperature in response to hot stimuli in the mouth who presents with confluent erythematous papules and pustules on the forehead, cheeks, and nose.
- There is an absence of comedones that are usually seen with acne.
- The peak incidence is 40 to 50 years and is more common in females.
- The lesions may last days to months.
- Treat by decreasing the patient's intake of hot beverages and using topical metronidazole gel.
- Oral antibiotics may be added.

Pityriasis Rosea
- *CLASSIC PRESENTATION:* A person who first has a single erythematous plaque with a scale in the central portion of the lesion, followed by a generalized eruption, classically in a "Christmas tree" distribution on the trunk, especially the back.
- This inflammation spontaneously resolves in 6 weeks.

Lupus Erythematosus
- *CLASSIC PRESENTATION:* A female in her thirties with bright red, erythematous plaques in a butterfly distribution on the face, often accompanied by fever, arthritis, renal, cardiac, or pulmonary disease.
- This illness is much more common in females and typically presents about the age of 30.
- There may be dark red, well-demarcated plaques on the dorsal aspects of the fingers and hands with sparing of the skin overlying the joints.
- The rash often involves sun-exposed areas.
- For further details, see the Internal Medicine chapter.

Psoriasis
- *CLASSIC PRESENTATION:* A person with chronic scaling plaques in characteristic sites of the body, which include extensor surfaces such as the elbows and knees as well as the scalp, intertriginous areas, and the soles of the feet.

- This is a hereditary disorder that is equally common in males and females.
- There is a bimodal age distribution of the teens/twenties and age fifties.
- The face is not commonly involved.
- Treat initially with topical corticosteroids.

PEDIATRIC DERMATOLOGY

Measles
- *CLASSIC PRESENTATION:* A child with a prodrome of malaise, fever, cough, coryza, conjunctivitis, and photophobia, followed by an erythematous maculopapular rash that begins on the head and spreads downward.
- Koplik's spots on the buccal mucosa are pathognomonic (small red spots with central gray specks).
- The diagnosis is made by clinical findings and therapy is supportive.
- Vitamin A supplementation should be given for patients between the ages of 6 months and 2 years who require hospitalization.

Roseola Infantum
- *CLASSIC PRESENTATION:* A child with a high fever followed by a maculopapular rash on the trunk that spreads peripherally.
- Roseola infantum is caused by human herpes virus 6.
- There may be a high leukocyte count initially with a left shift.
- Leukopenia and neutropenia are seen by the second day.

Erythema Infectiosum (Fifth Disease)
- *CLASSIC PRESENTATION:* A child with a rash that begins as erythema of the cheeks with a "slapped cheek" appearance.
- Fifth disease is caused by parvovirus B-19.
- There is no prodrome.
- The erythematous maculopapular rash has a reticular (lacy) appearance and usually involves the arms and spreads to the trunk and legs.
- There is a low grade fever with fluctuation in severity of the rash.

Chickenpox (Varicella)
- *CLASSIC PRESENTATION:* A child with a prodrome of mild fever, malaise, and anorexia followed by the eruption of 1 to 2 mm vesicles on an erythematous base that are often described as a "dewdrop on a rose petal." The lesions are very pruritic.
- The lesions occur in crops, so there are lesions at several different stages of development.
- Patients are extremely infectious until all of the lesions are crusted.

Impetigo

- *CLASSIC PRESENTATION:* A child with small golden crusted lesions on the face, arms, legs, and buttocks.
- Impetigo is most commonly caused by *Staphylococcus aureus* and *Streptococcus pyogenes* (group A Strep).
- Primary impetigo arises at minor breaks in the skin.
- Treat with topical antibiotics.

Scarlet Fever

- *CLASSIC PRESENTATION:* A child with a characteristic erythematous "sandpaper" rash that blanches with pressure. The rash appears first on the wrists and ankles and then spreads to the trunk and quickly becomes generalized. Other signs of scarlet fever include circumoral pallor and a "strawberry tongue."
- The rash of scarlet fever is caused by streptococcal pyogenic exotoxins.
- Treat with penicillin.

Rocky Mountain Spotted Fever

- *CLASSIC PRESENTATION:* A child in the 5- to 9-year-old age group with the sudden onset of fever, headache, myalgias, mental confusion, and rash. The pink rash appears on day 3 to 5. Macules, which blanch on compression, first appear on the hands, wrists, feet, and ankles and spread to involve the entire body.
- There is often a history of a tick bite.
- This is a rare illness (approximately 6000 cases/year) caused the bite of ticks infected by *Rickettsia rickettsii.*
- Treat with chloramphenicol or tetracycline (which can stain the teeth of children less than 9 years old).

Scabies

- *CLASSIC PRESENTATION:* A child or young adult with an intensely pruritic rash with pustules and burrows.
- Scabies is caused by infestation by the mite *Sarcoptes scabiei.*
- The linear burrows are found most commonly in the folds between the fingers and toes.
- Scabies is spread by direct contact.
- It is usually diagnosed by clinical appearance.
- The treatment of choice is 5% permethrin topical ointment or oral ivermectin.

SKIN CANCERS

Basal Cell Carcinoma

- *CLASSIC PRESENTATION:* A person over age 40 with light skin and a history of sunlight exposure who presents with a pink or red translucent or "pearly" nodule.
- This is the most common type of skin cancer.

- The lesion appears most commonly on sun-exposed surfaces such as the ears, nose, and head.
- The nodule may be ulcerated with a rolled border.
- The shape is round or oval with a depressed center.
- This cancer is locally invasive and destructive, but has a limited metastatic potential.
- Treat with surgical excision.

Squamous Cell Carcinoma
- *CLASSIC PRESENTATION:* A patient with light skin and a history of sun exposure who presents with a slowly evolving a hyperkeratotic, scaly, ulcerated lesion in a sun-exposed area.
- This cancer is usually locally metastatic.
- Treat with surgical excision.

Melanoma
- *CLASSIC PRESENTATION:* A patient with light skin and a history of sun exposure who presents with an colored, raised, solitary lesion with irregular borders.
- There is usually a single lesion with tiny satellite lesions.
- There is often a family history of melanoma or a history of precursor lesions.
- The lesion usually evolves over 1 to 2 years.
- The lesion may be brown, blue, black, or red.
- Melanoma is usually highly malignant and can metastasize both locally and systemically.
- Remember the mnemonic ABCDE to help recognize melanoma:

  Asymmetry

  Border irregularity

  Color is mottled (mixed)

  Diameter > 6 mm

  Enlargement over time and Elevation
- Treat with excision with margins and biopsy.

NOTES

Chapter 10

RADIOLOGY

Theodore X. O'Connell, M.D.

HEAD RADIOLOGY

Multiple Myeloma

- *CLASSIC PRESENTATION:* Punched-out bony lesions seen in the skull with a "salt and pepper" appearance.
- Bone pain is the most common symptom and it usually is felt in the back or ribs.
- The next most common clinical problem is susceptibility to bacterial infections, especially pneumonias.
- Multiple myeloma is more common in older people and African Americans.
- The clinical syndrome can be recalled with the mnemonic PLASMA:

  Proteinuria/renal insufficiency
  Lytic bone lesions and hypercalcemia
  Anemia/Abnormal bleeding
  Sepsis and other infections
  Marrow involvement
  Amyloidosis

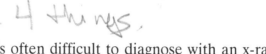

Basilar Skull Fracture

- Basilar skull fracture is often difficult to diagnose with an x-ray, but the following triad is virtually diagnostic:
  1. Periorbital ecchymoses (raccoon eyes)
  2. Postauricular ecchymoses (Battle's sign)
  3. Blood behind the tympanic membrane (hemotympanum)
- Otorrhea or rhinorrhea indicate cerebrospinal fluid leakage.

Brain Tumor

- *CLASSIC PRESENTATION:* A patient who presents with a history of neurological deficits, headache, new-onset seizure, vomiting, or altered mental status. A mass may be seen on CT scan or MRI of the brain with possible compression of adjacent intracerebral structures.
- A history of personality changes or seizures would suggest a mass in the temporal lobe.
- In adults, two thirds of brain tumors are supratentorial.
- In children, two thirds of brain tumors are infratentorial (kids=lower).
- In adults, metastatic neoplasms are the most common, followed by gliomas and meningiomas.
- In children, astrocytomas and medulloblastomas are the most common.

Subarachnoid Hemorrhage

- *CLASSIC PRESENTATION:* A patient with a complaint of "the worst headache of my life," and a CT scan showing subarachnoid blood.

- These are most often due to trauma or a ruptured berry aneurysm.

Subdural Hematoma
- *CLASSIC PRESENTATION:* A patient with a history of head trauma and a CT scan that shows a smooth, biconvex lens-shaped mass, often located over the lateral surface of the frontal or parietal lobes.
- The bleeding is due to laceration of subdural bridging veins.
- Altered mental status is often a prominent symptom.
- Treatment consists of evacuation of the clot.

Intracerebral Hemorrhage
- *CLASSIC PRESENTATION:* A patient with a history of hypertensive or atherosclerotic disease with new-onset stroke symptoms and a CT scan showing bleeding within the brain parenchyma.
- Bleeding can also be due to coagulopathies, tumor, or trauma.
- Common symptoms include hemiplegia and hemisensory deficits.
- Two thirds present with coma.
- Two thirds of the bleeding sites are in the basal ganglia.

CHEST RADIOLOGY

Tuberculosis
- *CLASSIC PRESENTATION:* A chest x-ray showing calcified or enlarged intrathoracic lymph nodes and a single cavitary lesion in a patient with a history of increasing cough, hemoptysis, fatigue, and weight loss.
- In addition to the lymph node changes, infiltrates in the posterior segment of the upper lobes, cavitary lesions, satellite lesions, volume loss in the upper lobes, and apical thickening may be seen.

Coccidioidomycosis (Valley Fever)
- *CLASSIC PRESENTATION:* A patient with a history of travel to the southwest United States and a chest x-ray showing a coin-like lesion or a single thin-walled cavitary lesion.
- Symptoms may range from a flu-like illness to severe pneumonia.

Pulmonary Embolus
- *CLASSIC PRESENTATION:* A patient with shortness of breath and pleuritic chest pain with a chest x-ray showing decreased pulmonary vascular markings in a wedge-shaped distribution (Westermark's sign).
- Other symptoms include tachypnea, hemoptysis, and hypotension.

- Arterial blood gas measurement shows decreased PO_2 and decreased PCO_2 (the decreased PCO_2 is due to hyperventilation).
- The diagnostic test of choice is a pulmonary angiogram, but VQ scan, spiral CT scan, or MRI may also be used.

Pneumonia

- *CLASSIC PRESENTATION:* A patient with a productive cough, fever, and chest pain with coughing, whose chest x-ray shows an infiltrate (an opaque area) that is most often focal.
- Other symptoms may include headache, myalgias, fatigue, sore throat, nausea, vomiting, and diarrhea.
- Physical examination often reveals rales, dullness to percussion, and bronchial breath sounds.
- If diarrhea is present, consider *Legionella*.
- A diffuse distribution of infiltrates suggests *Pneumocystis carinii*, CMV, measles, or herpes zoster viral infection.
- Histoplasmosis should also be suspected, especially if the patient has been living near the Ohio or Mississippi River Valley.
- Finally, fungal pneumonia should be considered in any immunocompromised or long-term hospitalized patient.
- A sputum examination is used to diagnose bacterial pneumonia.

Pneumothorax

- *CLASSIC PRESENTATION:* A patient with pleuritic chest pain and dyspnea with an x-ray showing a loss of vascular markings (often apical) with a water-density line medially that represents the visceral pleura covering the retracted lung apex.
- Tracheal deviation may be seen.
- Hyperresonance and decreased breath sounds are heard over the involved side.
- Spontaneous pneumothorax usually occurs in young, thin, tall males.
- Treatment usually consists of insertion of a chest tube to evacuate the air.

Lung Cancer

- *CLASSIC PRESENTATION:* A patient with a history of cough, hemoptysis, obstructive pneumonia, chest pain, hoarseness, or superior vena cava syndrome with a chest x-ray showing a coin lesion (solitary pulmonary nodule) greater than 1 cm, often with indistinct margins. Growth of the lesion may be seen on follow-up x-ray.
- Systemic symptoms may include anorexia and weight loss.
- There is often a history of tobacco smoking.

Sarcoidosis

- *CLASSIC PRESENTATION:* An African-American woman between the ages of 20 and 50 with fatigue, exertional dyspnea, nonproductive cough, and a chest x-ray showing bilateral hilar lymphadenopathy with or without pulmonary infiltrates.
- Noncaseating granulomas are the fundamental lesions, and they are most often located in the lungs.
- Cutaneous or ocular lesions are also frequent.
- Corticosteroids are the typical treatment of choice.

ABDOMINAL RADIOLOGY

Diverticula

- *CLASSIC PRESENTATION:* Diverticula are seen as small outpouchings from the colon on barium enema films in an individual over the age of 60.
- There may be a history of left lower quadrant abdominal pain with alternating diarrhea and constipation.
- Diverticula occur most often in the colon, especially the sigmoid colon.
- Diverticulitis may present with left lower quadrant abdominal pain, fever, and constipation. It is often called "left-sided appendicitis."
- Metronidazole and ciprofloxacin are the treatment of choice for diverticulitis.
- Symptoms may be reduced by increasing stool bulk with high-fiber foods.

Gallstones

- *CLASSIC PRESENTATION:* Cholecystitis presents with right upper quadrant abdominal pain/tenderness, fatty food intolerance, nausea, vomiting, referred right subscapular pain, and a positive Murphy's sign (acute pain and inspiratory arrest elicited by palpation of the right upper quadrant during inspiration).
- Only about 10% of gallstones are seen on an x-ray; therefore, ultrasound is the diagnostic study of choice.
- Gallstones are more common in patients with the five F's:

  Female
  Fat
  Forty
  Fertile (multiparity)
  Flatulent

- Right upper quadrant ultrasound in cholecystitis reveals a dilated gallbladder with stones, often with a dilated cystic duct. Also look for dilation of the common bile duct, indicating acute obstruction of bile flow.

Hirschsprung's Disease

- *CLASSIC PRESENTATION:* A barium enema showing a narrowed, diseased distal colon and rectum with a dilated, normal proximal colon.
- Hirschsprung's disease is due to the congenital lack of enteric ganglia of the distal colon and rectum, leading to dilation of the proximal colon.
- A full-thickness rectal biopsy reveals the absence of enteric ganglia.

Kidney Stones

- Ninety percent of kidney stones may be seen on abdominal x-ray.
- There is often a history of flank pain, testicular pain, and hematuria.
- Calcium oxalate stones are the most common.
- Struvite stones are found only in the presence of a urinary tract infection.

Viscus Perforation

- *CLASSIC PRESENTATION:* A patient with a history of acute abdominal symptoms or ulcerative disease whose abdominal x-ray reveals free intraperitoneal air outlining the diaphragm or liver.

EXTREMITY RADIOLOGY

Colles' Fracture

- *CLASSIC PRESENTATION:* A patient who has had a fall onto an outstretched hand who complains of wrist or arm pain.
- An x-ray will show a fracture of the distal radius.
- Treatment consists of reduction and immobilization.

Scaphoid Fracture

- *CLASSIC PRESENTATION:* A patient who has had an injury to the hand or wrist and has tenderness over the anatomical snuff box on physical examination.
- An x-ray may show a fracture of the scaphoid bone, but often is negative. If it is negative, the x-ray should be repeated in a few weeks.
- This is the most common fracture of the carpal bones.
- Treat with immobilization.

Spiral Fracture

- Any spiral fracture in a long bone of a child should raise the suspicion of child abuse since the fracture is caused by the twisting motion of an extremity.

Femoral Neck Fracture

- *CLASSIC PRESENTATION:* An older woman who has had a fall and presents with groin or hip pain and limited movement in one of her hips. An x-ray of the hip shows a fracture most often through the femoral neck.
- There is a risk of avascular necrosis, so rapid treatment is necessary.
- Treat with open fixation.

Slipped Capital Femoral Epiphysis

- *CLASSIC PRESENTATION:* An obese pubescent male with hip or knee pain and a radiograph of the hip showing an "ice cream falling off the cone," which represents the displacement of the femoral head off the femoral metaphysis.
- This displacement can occur in the absence of any known physical trauma.
- The patient also frequently has an altered gait and limited range of motion in the affected hip.
- Treat with surgical fixation.

Osteosarcoma

- *CLASSIC PRESENTATION:* A male between 10 and 20 years old with a bony growth in an area around the knee and an x-ray showing new bone formation in the affected area. Classically there is periosteal elevation and a "sunburst" pattern of soft tissue calcification.
- This is the most common bone tumor in children.
- Two thirds of these tumors occur near the knees in either the distal femur or proximal tibia.
- Treat with surgical resection and chemotherapy.

ARTERIOGRAPHY

Carotid Artery Stenosis

- *CLASSIC PRESENTATION:* An older patient with a history of transient ischemic attack or amaurosis fugax (transient blindness) who has a carotid angiogram showing an area of narrowing.
- The lesion is due to atherosclerosis and most often occurs in the area of the bifurcation of the carotid artery in the neck.
- Cervical bruits may be heard on physical examination.
- The territory of the middle cerebral artery is most often affected.
- Treatment with carotid endarterectomy has been shown to be most efficacious.

NOTES

Chapter 11

OPHTHALMOLOGY

Susan L. Taylor, M.D.

Conjunctivitis

- *CLASSIC PRESENTATION:* A patient with blurry vision, tearing, and discharge with conjunctival erythema and edema. The blurred vision clears with blinking.
- In neonates, it is usually caused by *Staphylococcus*, *Gonococcus*, or *Chlamydia*. Use prophylactic silver nitrate, tetracycline, or erythromycin for gonococcal prophylaxis.
- In adults, adenovirus is the leading cause of conjunctivitis. The course is usually self-limited and benign. In general, viral conjunctivitis usually causes a clear ocular discharge, whereas bacterial conjunctivitis more often causes a pus-like discharge.
- Ocular antibiotics are given when there is any suspicion of bacterial conjunctivitis to prevent abscess formation. If conjunctivitis does not improve with antibiotics, herpes simplex virus should be suspected, and can be visualized with fluorescein.

Keratitis

- *CLASSIC PRESENTATION:* A patient with ocular pain, blurry vision, photophobia, tearing, conjunctival erythema and edema.
- Look for inflammation or ulceration of the cornea on slit lamp examination.

Uveitis

- *CLASSIC PRESENTATION:* A patient with ocular pain, photophobia, and blurred vision with conjunctival erythema. The symptoms are similar to those of keratitis, but there are different findings on ocular examination. Ocular examination reveals inflammation of uveal structures such as the iris, ciliary body, or choroid in any combination.
- The cause is usually idiopathic.
- Treat with cycloplegic drops and glucocorticoids.

Cataract

- *CLASSIC PRESENTATION:* An older patient with blurred vision, visual glare, altered color perception, and monocular diplopia.
- A cataract is an opacification of the lens that develops over months to years. There may be a history of sun exposure without eye protection.
- Treat with surgical cataract removal.

Central Retinal Artery Occlusion

- *CLASSIC PRESENTATION:* Sudden painless vision loss in one eye.
- If vision loss resolves in minutes, this is known as a type of transient ischemic attack (TIA) called amaurosis fugax. If the occlusion is persistent, it results in infarction of the neural retina, and permanent blindness can result.
- On examination, the retina is pale with a cherry-red spot at the macula.
- Temporal arteritis should be ruled out (see Neurology chapter).
- This is an ophthalmologic emergency. An ophthalmologist may attempt to move embolic material into peripheral arterioles.

Acute Glaucoma (Angle-Closure Glaucoma)

- *CLASSIC PRESENTATION:* A patient with sudden onset blurred vision in one eye, accompanied by excruciating ocular pain.
- The increased intraocular pressure results from the decreased outflow of aqueous humor through the pupil, trabecular network, and Schlemm's canal.
- On examination there is increased intraocular pressure, but no papilledema.
- Treatment consists of the reduction of intraocular pressure with the use of hyperosmotic agents such as mannitol. Parenteral acetazolamide and topical pilocarpine may also be used. Surgery may be required.

Chronic Glaucoma (Open-Angle Glaucoma)

- *CLASSIC PRESENTATION:* A patient with painless, slow loss of peripheral and paracentral visual fields.
- Elevated intraocular pressure causes damage to the optic nerve, resulting in the loss of peripheral and paracentral visual fields.
- Chronic glaucoma is treated with pilocarpine, β-adrenergic blockers (timolol), and sympathomimetics (epinephrine). Carbonic anhydrase inhibitors (acetazolamide) may also be used.

Optic Neuritis

- *CLASSIC PRESENTATION:* A 20- to 30-year-old patient with unilateral vision loss and ocular pain that worsens with movement.
- Upon examination, there is a relative afferent pupillary defect. Papilledema is diagnostic.
- Multiple sclerosis is the leading cause of this condition. Optic neuritis is also harbinger of multiple sclerosis.
- Treat with methylprednisolone.

Increased Intracranial Pressure

- *CLASSIC PRESENTATION:* A patient with papilledema without visual changes, sometimes with photophobia. Other signs of increased intracranial pressure, e.g., nausea, vomiting, and headache, may be present.
- If there are abnormal CSF or radiological findings indicating infection, tumor, or hemorrhage, this is an emergency!
- Pseudotumor cerebri (also known as benign intracranial hypertension) is a condition classically occurring in young, overweight women, in which there is gross papilledema with increased intracranial pressure. CSF analysis and radiologic films are normal. The cause is most often idiopathic, but may be associated with vitamin A excess.
- Initial treatment is head elevation, hyperventilation, fluid restriction, hyperosmotic agents (mannitol), and a diuretic.

Retinal Detachment

- *CLASSIC PRESENTATION:* Painless monocular vision loss, often related to head trauma.
- On physical examination, the detached portion of the retina looks like a gray cloud.
- Emergency surgery is required to save the retina.

Chapter 12

STATISTICS

Theodore X. O'Connell, M.D.

Table 12.1 below will facilitate defining several clinically useful terms.

	Disease present	Disease absent
Test positive	*a* (true positives)	*b* (false positives)
Test negative	*c* (false negatives)	*d* (true negatives)

Sensitivity

- Sensitivity $= \dfrac{a}{a + c}$

- Sensitivity $= \dfrac{\textit{patients with disease and positive test}}{\textit{all patients with disease}}$

- Sensitivity is defined as the probability that a test result will be positive when administered to patients who have the disease.
- A test with high sensitivity has few false negatives.
- A screening test should have a high sensitivity to minimize the number of false negative test results.

Specificity

- Specificity $= \dfrac{d}{b + d}$

- Specificity $= \dfrac{\textit{patients with no disease and negative test}}{\textit{all patients with no disease}}$

- Specificity is defined as the probability that a test result will be negative when administered to patients without the disease.
- A test with high specificity has few false positives.
- Tests used to verify the presence of disease should have a high specificity to minimize the number of false positive test results.

Positive Predictive Value

- Positive Predictive Value = $\dfrac{a}{a + b}$

- Positive predictive value = $\dfrac{\textit{true positive patients}}{\textit{all positive patients}}$

- Positive predictive value is the probability that a patient with a positive screening test actually has the disease.
- The positive predictive value increases when the prevalence of a disease increases.

Negative Predictive Value

- Negative Predictive Value = $\dfrac{d}{c + d}$

- Negative predictive value = $\dfrac{\textit{true negative patients}}{\textit{all negative patients}}$

- Negative predictive value is the probability that a patient with a negative screening test result actually does not have the disease.

Lead Time Bias
- Lead time bias is the seemingly improved disease survival from screening tests for disease. The increased survival time is due to earlier detection of the disease and not necessarily to increased survival time.
- For example, when a patient undergoes a screening test for a serious disease and has a positive result, his disease is diagnosed earlier than it would have been had the screening test not been done. However, if the early detection of the disease does not result in more effective therapy for the disease, the patient gains nothing and knows for a longer time that the untreatable disease is present.
- In essence, the screening detection of a disease may appear to increase the survival time because the disease was detected earlier, but in reality the screening test does not affect the course of the patient's disease.

Prevalence
- Prevalence is the number of cases present at a single moment in time.

- Prevalence is higher than incidence for long-term illness such as hypertension since there are more patients with hypertension at any given time than there are new cases diagnosed in a year.

Incidence

- Incidence is the number of new cases in a given period of time (often 1 year).
- Incidence is higher than prevalence for short-term illnesses such as pneumonia since there are more cases diagnosed in a year than there are at any given time.
- When the observed incidence greatly exceeds the expected incidence of a disease, an epidemic is present.

Reliability

- Reliability is the ability of a test to be reproduced.

Validity

- Validity is how well a test actually measures what it is supposed to measure.

Odds Ratio

Table 12.2 can be used to define odds ratio.

	Disease present	Disease absent
+ Exposure	*a*	*b*
- Exposure	*c*	*d*

- Odds ratio = $\dfrac{a \times d}{b \times c}$

- The odds ratio approximates the relative risk of disease in an exposed group compared with an unexposed group. The odds ratio is used in retrospective (case-control) studies.

INDEX OF CLASSIC PRESENTATIONS

, renal cell, 86
, squamous cell, 189
, thyroid, 95
, transitional cell, 86
cardiomyopathy, dilated, 107
, hypertrophic, 107
, restrictive, 107
cataract, 200
chickenpox, 187
cholelithiasis, 133
coccidioidomycosis, 193
colitis, ulcerative, 141
concussion, 163
conjunctivitis, 200
cough, whooping, 11
crisis, hypertensive, 102
croup, 10
cysts, functional ovarian, 57

D
deficiency, factor VIII, 19
, niacin, 67
, thiamine, 67
, total parenteral nutrition-related, 68
, vitamin A, 68
, vitamin B_1, 67
, vitamin B_6, 67
, vitamin C, 67
, vitamin D, 68
, vitamin E, 68
, vitamin K, 68
degeneration, hepatolenticular, 91
delirium, 169
dementia, 169
dependence, stimulant, 173
, substance, 173
depression, major, 166
dermatitis, contact, 186
detachment, retinal, 202
diabetes, insipidus, 93
, mellitus, 96-97
, gestational, 33
disease, Addison's, 96
, alcoholic liver, 91

209

G-H

I-L

M-O

neuroblastoma, 21
neurofibromatosis, 76
obstruction, small bowel, 131
occlusion, central retinal artery, 200
osteoarthritis, 69
osteosarcoma, 197
otitis externa, 7
otitis media, 7

P-R
pancreatitis, acute, 134
       , chronic, 135
pellagra, 67
perforation, viscus, 196
pericarditis, acute, 108
       , chronic, 108
       , constrictive, 108
phenylketonuria, 26
pityriasis rosea, 186
placenta previa, 40
poisoning, methanol, 98
     , methylene glycol, 98
polycythemia vera, 72
polyposis, familial adenomatous, 138
polyps, colonic, 138
pneumonia, 194
      , aspiration, 82
      , atypical, 81
      , chlamydial, 6
      , classical bacterial, 81
      , mycoplasma, 6
pneumothorax, 115, 194
       , spontaneous, 78
preeclampsia/eclampsia, 34
pregnancy, ectopic, 37
pressure, elevated intracranial, 162, 201
pseudogout, 69
pseudotumor cerebri, 156
psoriasis, 186
purpura, idiopathic thrombocytopenic, 22
    , Henoch-Schönlein, 22
pyelonephritis, 14
rickets, 68
rosacea, 186

213

roseola infantum, 187
rupture, uterine, 42

S

sarcoidosis, 79, 195
sarcoma, Ewing's, 22
    , osteogenic, 22
scabies, 188
schizophrenia, 171
sclerosis, multiple, 160
scoliosis, 5
scurvy, 67
seizures, febrile, 8
sinusitis, acute, 7
sepsis, neonatal, 6
SLE, 70
stenosis, carotid artery, 197
    , pyloric, 12
strep throat, 6
stroke, 156
    , hemorrhagic, 157
    , thromboembolic, 157
    , thrombotic, 157
syndrome, acquired immunodeficiency, 82
    , acute respiratory distress, 78
    , Alport's, 85
    , Boerhaave's, 128
    , carcinoid, 92
    , compartment, 149
    , Cushing's, 96
    , Down's, 23
    , Edwards', 24
    , fragile X, 26
    , Goodpasture's, 79
    , Guillain-Barré, 9
    , inappropriate ADH release, 94
    , Klinefelter's, 25
    , Lambert-Eaton, 161
    , Mallory-Weiss, 128
    , Marfan's, 24, 75
    , MEN, 95
    , mucocutaneous lymph node, 23
    , nephritic, 15
    , nephrotic, 14

Other USMLE, Step 2 Review Books
Available from J & S Publishing Company, Inc.

Surgery: Review for New National Boards
Glenn W. Geelhoed, MD, FACS
ISBN 0-9632873-5-4, 246 pp., $ 25.00
Extensively illustrated with black and white clinical case examples. Trade Paperback, 562 practice test items with answers and explanatory tutorials. This is an abridged version of *The Study of Surgery*.

The Study of Surgery
Glenn W. Geelhoed, MD, FACS
ISBN 0-9632873-6-2, 392 pp., $ 40.00
Extensively illustrated with full color and black and white clinical case examples. Trade Paperback, 1060 test items with answers and explanatory tutorials. Special section of strategies for passing multiple choice examinations.

PLEASE NOTE: You won't want both Surgery books because *The Study of Surgery* includes everything found in *Surgery: Review for New National Boards* plus color pictures, an additional 498 items, and a section on passing strategies for USMLE, Step 2 examinations. We suggest that you buy the more comprehensive book entitled *The Study of Surgery*.

Obstetrics and Gynecology: Review for New National Boards
Ralph L. Kramer, MD, FACOG
ISBN 0-9632873-9-7, 190 pp., $ 25.00
Extensively illustrated with black and white clinical case examples. Trade Paperback, 530 practice test items with answers and explanatory tutorials.

These books are available at your **LOCAL MEDICAL BOOKSTORE.** We urge you to purchase these books there. If you do not have access to a medical bookstore, our books are also available from www.lb.com, www.amazon.com, www.medbookstore.com, www.barnesandnoble.com, and www.discountmedicalbooks.com, using a credit card. If all else fails, you can order direct from the publisher by mailing a personal check, money order, or cash (sorry no credit cards). Please remit cost of book(s) plus $ 3.20/book for shipping and handling (our cost) to:

Order Department
J & S Publishing Company, Inc.
1300 Bishop Lane
Alexandria, VA 22302 USA

e-mail jandspub@ix.netcom.com
URL http://www.jandspub.com
Phone 703-823-9833
Fax   703-823-9834

We will ship books via USPS Priority Mail within 24 hours of receipt of your check, money order, or cash. Good luck on your examinations.